Praise for Controlling Your Drinking

"In a nonjudgmental way, this book helps you scope out your issues with alcohol and decide what to do, putting the ball in your court instead of being prescriptive. It is filled with useful and practical strategies that you can pick and choose from to meet your own needs."
—Anne M. Fletcher, author of *Inside Rehab* and *Sober for Good*

"Clear, concise, nonjudgmental and practical, it lays out the facts that are often obscured in the heated debate over alcohol treatments....Offers tools for successful moderation...as well as tactics for dealing with common challenges."
—*Publishers Weekly*

"Now in its second edition, this book has only gotten better. By helping readers overcome alcohol problems on their own, this book fills an enormous need, and is consistent with the scientific evidence that self-change is a common pathway to recovery. A welcome alternative in a field where those with concerns about their alcohol use are given few options."
—Linda Carter Sobell, PhD, ABPP, and Mark B. Sobell, PhD, ABPP, Center for Psychological Studies, Nova Southeastern University

"The authors provide excellent advice and suggestions....Throughout are numerous practical tools and techniques that anyone can grasp....Highly recommended."
—*Library Journal*

"Drs. Miller and Muñoz provide an easy-to-follow approach for people who are worried they may be drinking too much. The tools presented here for achieving moderate drinking are supported by a wealth of evidence; examples sprinkled throughout the book illustrate how to accomplish each goal of the program. Anyone who has struggled with the need to cut down will benefit from reading this book and following its simple, honest advice."
—Katie Witkiewitz, PhD, Department of Psychology, University of New Mexico

Controlling Your Drinking

Other Titles from William R. Miller

For General Readers

Quantum Change:
When Epiphanies and Sudden Insights Transform Ordinary Lives
William R. Miller and Janet C'de Baca

For Professionals

Motivational Interviewing (3rd ed.): Helping People Change
William R. Miller and Stephen Rollnick

Motivational Interviewing in Health Care:
Helping Patients Change Behavior
Stephen Rollnick, William R. Miller, and Christopher C. Butler

Motivational Interviewing in the Treatment of Psychological Problems
*Edited by Hal Arkowitz, Henny A. Westra, William R. Miller,
and Stephen Rollnick*

Controlling Your Drinking

Tools to Make Moderation Work for You

SECOND EDITION

William R. Miller, PhD

Ricardo F. Muñoz, PhD

THE GUILFORD PRESS

New York   London

© 2013 The Guilford Press
A Division of Guilford Publications, Inc.
72 Spring Street, New York, NY 10012
www.guilford.com

The information in this volume is not intended as a substitute for consultation with healthcare professionals. Each individual's health concerns should be evaluated by a qualified professional.

Printed in the United States of America

This book is printed on acid-free paper.

Last digit is print number: 9   8   7   6   5   4   3   2   1

Library of Congress Cataloging-in-Publication Data

Miller, William R. (William Richard)
    Controlling your drinking : tools to make moderation work for you / William R.
  Miller and Ricardo F. Muñoz. — Second edition.
        pages   cm
    Includes bibliographical references and index.
    ISBN 978-1-4625-0759-7 (pbk.: alk. paper) — ISBN 978-1-4625-1045-0 (hardcover:
  alk. paper)
      1. Controlled drinking.   2. Alcoholism.   3. Self-care, Health.
  I. Muñoz, Ricardo F.   II. Title.
    HV5278.M55 2013
    613.81—dc23

                                              2013011366

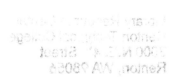

To the pioneers:
Syd Lovibond, Mark and Linda Sobell,
and Alan Marlatt
—WRM

To Clara Luz and Luis Alberto,
and to Pat, Rodrigo, and Aubrey
—RFM

Contents

Preface   ix

Acknowledgments   xi

PART I   Introduction

   1   Thinking about Drinking   3

   2   Why Change?   11

   3   Is Moderation for You?   20

PART II   When You Drink

   4   Getting Started   35

   5   Keeping Track   55

   6   Taking Charge   67

   7   Slowing Down   70

   8   Refusing Drinks   79

   9   Affirming Your Progress   83

  10   Moving Along   95

PART III   Before You Drink

  11   Discovering Your Triggers   101

  12   Places   104

  13   People   108

  14   Days and Times   112

  15   Feelings   115

16   Other Triggers   120

17   Summary: Before You Drink   126

PART IV   Instead of Drinking

18   Relaxing   135

19   Self-Talk   143

20   Pleasant Activities without Alcohol   149

21   Coping with Negative Moods and Depression   155

22   Self-Concept   168

23   Sleeping Well   177

24   Mindfulness   184

25   Managing Anxiety and Fear   193

26   Being Assertive   203

27   Relating to Others   209

28   Living "As If"   218

PART V   How Are You Doing?

29   If Moderation Isn't Working for You   225

30   Sources of Help   234

Appendix A   The Wrath of Grapes: Reasons for Concern   243

Appendix B   An Inventory of Alcohol-Related Problems   249

Appendix C   Tables for Estimating Blood Alcohol   251
                      Concentration (BAC)

Going Further: Recommended Resources   269

Notes   273

Bibliography   277

Index   283

About the Authors   290

Purchasers may download and print select practical
tools from this book at *www.guilford.com/p/miller7.*

Preface

How people think about drinking and related problems has changed substantially since we first published a book on controlling drinking in 1976. Back then, both popular and professional thinking was that there are two kinds of people in the world: alcoholics and nonalcoholics. The assumption was that if you're an alcoholic then you're incapable of controlling your drinking, and if you're not then you can drink as you please and have nothing to worry about. In other words, "alcoholics" can't control their drinking and other people don't need to!

Four decades later, there is much greater consciousness of the health and social consequences of heavy drinking. We are also collectively more aware of risks related to even a single occasion of overdrinking. Driving while intoxicated (DWI) continues to be a huge problem, but it has become much less socially acceptable and DWI-related fatalities in the United States have decreased by half. Physicians are now urged to ask routinely about patients' alcohol use and to advise heavy drinkers to reduce their consumption to low-risk levels. Alcohol use has become a health consideration like cholesterol, blood pressure, exercise, and body mass. Indeed, average alcohol consumption in America has dropped by half since it peaked in the 1960s.

It is still the case that some people who have been heavy drinkers find it best or easiest just to abstain from alcohol, and they have plenty of company. About one-third of adults in the United States now don't drink at all. As reflected in Chapter 3, we are also more able now to predict who will be successful in moderating their drinking. Ultimately what you choose to do about your own alcohol use is your decision. We hope that this book will be helpful in thinking it through.

The information and advice that we offer here is based on a long series of clinical studies begun in the 1970s. Our goal was to find better ways to help people manage their drinking and prevent alcohol-related health and social problems. We tried some complicated methods and some simpler ones, and across 20 years of randomized trials we found that people on average reduced their consumption by half or more. (The stories you'll read in this book were informed by the experiences of many of these people, although all identifying details have been changed and many anecdotes are composites of typical experiences we have come across again and again.) Happily, the simpler methods worked as well as the more complex (and expensive) ones, and there was another surprise. As a comparison condition we always included a group who after initial consultation received a copy of this book and went home to work at it on their own. They were just as successful on average in controlling their drinking as were those who were working with a counselor. In retrospect this should not have been surprising, because ultimately change is self-change.

So that is why four decades later we are still revising and updating this book as an evidence-based self-help method for managing your drinking. There are no guarantees, of course, and merely reading this book isn't likely to make much difference. What you will find in the chapters that follow is our best current advice for those who want to control their drinking. You're the only person who can decide whether and how this approach will work for you.

Acknowledgments

In publishing the first guidebook to help people moderate their drinking, we built on the work of many colleagues whose research contributed to scientific knowledge about self-management. Our earliest clinical trials, which preceded our 1976 book, were inspired by the pioneering work of Syd Lovibond in Australia and that of Roger Vogler and Mark and Linda Sobell in the United States. Important early encouragement and expertise were provided by Robert Hall, Edward Lichtenstein, G. Alan Marlatt, John Marquis, Peter Miller, and Peter Nathan. Martha Sanchez-Craig conducted a meticulous series of clinical studies in Canada, spanning a three-decade research career. Important research and scholarship on this topic were contributed by many colleagues, including Lynn Alden, Tim Baker, Gerard Connors, Nick Heather, Reid Hester, and Ian Robertson. Psychology students at the University of New Mexico likewise contributed significantly to this research over the years, including Cheryl Taylor, Louise Baca, Lloyd Crawford, Kay Buck Harris, Rick Graber, Mark Joyce, Michael Markham, Dan Matthews, Martha Tinkcom, and JoAnne Cisneros West. Harold Delaney, Lane Leckman, and Edward Reyes brought critical conservatism to our methodology and analyses to help ensure that our findings were not overstated or misleading.

The technical production and improvement of our work was greatly aided by the editorial staff at The Guilford Press, including Kitty Moore, Chris Benton, and Jim Nageotte. What a pleasure it is to work with such helpful and competent people, who are as committed as their authors to producing a book that is both readable and effective. Muchas gracias!

Part I

•

Introduction

1

●

Thinking about Drinking

Many people drink alcohol, and most of them never experience serious harm or problems from doing it. Many others, however, do find at some point in their lives that their drinking is becoming risky or creating problems, and so they decide to cut down or quit. Some find that they need help to do so and seek professional consultation or attend mutual-help groups such as Alcoholics Anonymous. Many others cut down or quit drinking on their own.

Perhaps you're reading this book because you wonder whether you're drinking too much and ought to cut back. Problems related to drinking rarely spring up overnight, but rather build up gradually over a period of months or years. Often family members or others become concerned well before the drinker him- or herself does. Judging from our four decades of research, if you (or a loved one) are wondering whether you might be drinking too much, there is probably good reason for concern.

This book provides step-by-step guidance for deciding how much you will drink and then for reaching your chosen goal. The research-tested methods that we offer here are the best we know to help you moderate your drinking. We also offer suggestions for how to proceed if you find you have difficulty maintaining moderation, including the option of not consuming alcohol at all.

Overdrinking, Dumb Drinking, Harmful Drinking, and Dependent Drinking

Why is it that it can take so long for people to realize they're drinking too much and to do something about it? One obstacle, we believe, has been the

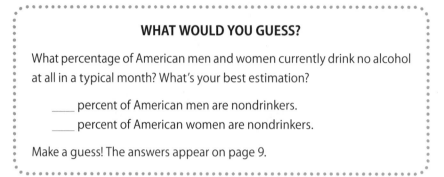

WHAT WOULD YOU GUESS?

What percentage of American men and women currently drink no alcohol at all in a typical month? What's your best estimation?

____ percent of American men are nondrinkers.

____ percent of American women are nondrinkers.

Make a guess! The answers appear on page 9.

label "alcoholic." When this term came into prominence a century ago, the belief emerged that either you are an alcoholic or you aren't: if you are, then there's nothing you can do about it except to stop drinking; and if you aren't, then you have nothing to worry about and can drink as much as you please. Furthermore, because "alcoholic" is a sticky label that carries a lot of social stigma. People tend to resent it and often endure many harsh consequences of overdrinking rather than accepting the label. Consequently, they take no action until their situation becomes very serious indeed.

This was pretty much the public view of alcoholism when the ideas in this book first saw print in 1976. Within that understanding, there would be no one to use a book like this: If you are alcoholic, then it's too late for moderation. If you're not alcoholic, then you don't need it. Or so popular thinking went at the time.

A lot more is known now about the many ways in which overdrinking can harm your physical, psychological, spiritual, and family health. If you're interested, Appendix A briefly summarizes current scientific reasons to be careful about alcohol. It is also clearer now just how many people are experiencing personal harm from their drinking. Those who fit the common stereotype of alcoholism account for only a small minority of alcohol-related health and social problems. They are but the tip of an immense iceberg.

In any event, we're not focused on labels here. We offer no slick test to tell you whether you "are" or "aren't." Instead, we want to help you think objectively about your drinking and how it may affect you.

Overdrinking

Perhaps the most common question is simply whether you drink *too much*. At relatively low levels of use, alcohol has no harmful effects for most people and may even offer some health benefits. Drinking above these safe limits, however, results in a rather steep increase in the rates and risk of a host of health and social problems. If your drinking exceeds safe limits, it may be termed "risky" or "hazardous," even if you have not yet experienced any significant negative consequences. We prefer the term "overdrinking" for its parallel to the term "overeating." "Overdrinking" applies only to the level or amount of drinking and does not imply the presence of any harm, problems, or dependence. It applies equally to a man who most days has a six pack of "light" beer between work and bedtime, a woman who drinks a bottle of wine once or twice a week, and the person whose daily fare is a fifth of scotch.

So how much is too much? The U.S. National Institutes of Health have recommended limits of one drink per day for women and two drinks per day for men.[1] (We will define what "one drink" means in Chapter 4.) A further general recommendation is not to drink every day but to give your body a rest from alcohol on at least one or two days a week.

Wow! Only one or two drinks a day? You may view that as an incredibly small amount of alcohol. Yet there are good reasons for these medically recommended limits. For most of the health problems described in Appendix A, risk levels are no different at zero, one, or two drinks per day. Above that level, however, risks for cancers, hypertension, stroke, and heart disease climb significantly: the more drinks per day, the higher the risk of serious health problems.[2]

These are just averages, of course. Most people who gamble do lose money, and a very few win big. That is why gambling establishments are so profitable. In the same way, the more you overdrink, the more likely you are to "lose" by developing significant physical, emotional, or social problems. A few people are fortunate and become that uncle or aunt, hero or grandparent who drank like a parched horse (or smoked two packs of cigarettes a day, or ate bacon cheeseburgers and butter-fried eggs all the time) for decades and still died at a ripe old age. It happens. As any life insurance actuary knows, however, mortality prediction statistics are dauntingly accurate for all of us collectively, even though it's more difficult to predict the longevity of any one particular person. Like smoking or overeating, overdrinking shortens life by as much as 10 to 15 years on average and can also detract greatly from quality-of-life years through disability, chronic disease, mental impairment, and harm done to family and other relationships.

Overdrinking shortens life by as much as 10 to 15 years.

One problem here is that these various outcomes

are probabilities. It is not *certain* that if you overdrink it will harm you or cause your premature death. It only *might* do so. If you knew for certain that the very next drink would kill you, chances are you wouldn't take it, but it's not that simple. Sustained heavy drinking (or smoking or overeating) will have dreadful consequences for some, some negative consequences for most, and no negative outcomes for some proportion of people during their lifetimes. Because there is no way to know for sure ahead of time which of these three groups would be yours, it's a matter of deciding which of the many available risks in life you choose to take.

Dumb Drinking

Certain kinds of harm do not require years of excess but can occur with a single occasion of overdrinking. Many of these have to do with drinking too much for conditions. What may be a reasonably safe amount of alcohol in one situation can have tragic results under other circumstances. In plain language, this is dumb drinking.

A classic example is drinking before driving. Even relatively small amounts of alcohol can subtly impair perception, judgment, attention, and other mental functions that are crucial for safe driving. The trouble, of course, is that it is hard to perceive when your perception is impaired or to judge when your judgment has been compromised. In the United States, the legal limit that defines "drunk" driving has declined over the years from 0.15 to 0.10, and now 0.08 g% (grams of alcohol per 100 milliliters [ml] of blood). Even at these lowered levels, however, there is clear impairment of the complex skills needed for safe driving. Other nations have made it illegal to drive at 0.02 or 0.03 g%, and scientific evidence shows reduction in alcohol-related fatalities when impaired-driving laws enforce these lower limits.

Certain kinds of harm can occur with a single occasion of overdrinking.

The only truly safe level of alcohol in the bloodstream when driving is *zero*. Our counsel is that if you are going to be driving, plan any drinking so that the alcohol has been *completely* eliminated from your body before you start the engine. In Chapter 4, we show you how to do this.

The only truly safe level of alcohol in the bloodstream when driving is zero.

Driving isn't the only activity that can be dangerously impaired by even moderate drinking. In search of a Christmas tree, one of our graduate students headed off to the mountains equipped with a chain saw. He felt completely unaffected by the two beers he drank while searching for the perfect tree, but with a small misjudgment he narrowly escaped cutting off his toes. Flying an airplane, swimming or boating, skiing, or using power tools—these are just a few examples of situations in which any drinking is hazardous. It takes only one such occasion to trigger a tragedy, and the newspapers are filled with them every year.

Rapid-paced drinking—such as occurs in drinking games, contests, or hazing—is another example of dumb drinking. It overrides normal judgment about how much is too much and opens the door for foolish risk taking.

Unfortunately, dumb drinking can take an almost infinite number of forms. Drinking before or during certain social situations holds potential for harm. For example, a substantial majority of date rapes occur when one or both people are under the influence of alcohol, a fact that also holds for other kinds of physical violence. Under the influence of alcohol, people are generally more likely to take risks, to do or say things that they wouldn't if sober, sometimes with long-lasting consequences, embarrassment, or guilt. Again, it's a matter of probabilities. On any one occasion of drinking, the chances of a tragic outcome are usually quite small. The trouble is, it can take only one instance of dumb drinking to change a life forever.

With rapid drinking, there is also a very real risk of dying from alcohol overdose. It is possible to drink enough to stop breathing, and this risk increases when combining alcohol with certain other drugs. The lethal dose level varies and can be much lower for children and youth.

Harmful Drinking

A third question to ask yourself, beyond how much you drink and in what potentially risky situations you drink, is the extent to which alcohol may already be causing problems or otherwise harming you or those around you. There are various inventories of the troubles that can pile up over time in relation to overdrinking. There is one in Chapter 3, and we've included a longer one in Appendix B. If you're on the fence as to whether you need to do anything about your drinking, an honest self-evaluation with these questionnaires can help you tally up the ways in which drinking may be causing harm, or at least starting to do so. Information is also provided in Appendix B to let you compare yourself with people seeking professional help for alcohol problems. If, on the other hand, you already know that your drinking is causing harm to you or others, there may be no particular need to visit Appendix B.

Harmful drinking has also sometimes been called "problem drinking" or "alcohol abuse," terms that can get in the way of taking an honest look at yourself. With regard to the first, people sometimes get hung up on whether they "have a drinking problem." What matters is not whether you merit a label, but rather what is happening in your life with regard to drinking and what, if anything, you choose to do about it. Alcohol "abuse" sounds both moralistic and odd. "Alcohol abuse," one witty colleague quipped, "is mixing single-malt scotch with root beer." We prefer the term "harmful drinking" because it describes exactly what is happening: it is drinking in a way that causes or contributes to harm.

Dependent Drinking

Finally, there is the concept of alcohol dependence. Some people think of this as being unable to stop drinking without suffering symptoms of alcohol withdrawal: shakiness, sweating, rapid heartbeat, and such. To be sure, it's possible to become physically addicted to alcohol in this way, but alcohol dependence is much larger than withdrawal. Many alcohol-dependent people do not feel shaky or sick when they stop drinking.

In the broadest sense, dependence is the process whereby a drug (in this case alcohol) gradually takes over more and more of your life. You spend more money buying alcohol, more time drinking and recovering from its effects. Consequently, people and activities with which you once spent more time begin to fall away. You spend more time with heavier drinkers and less time in places where there is no alcohol. Perhaps the idea of a party without alcohol makes you uncomfortable or just seems "inconvenient." You're not sure how you would deal with certain situations without alcohol, such as getting to sleep or feeling frustrated or down. From time to time you make an attempt to cut down or quit, but rather quickly go back to the familiar pattern. In short, alcohol slowly becomes central to your life.

A Word about Labels

Some people react so negatively to labels such as "problem drinker" and "alcoholic" that they avoid taking an honest look at what is actually happening to them. If you haven't noticed already, we are careful not to use such labels for people. We talk about harmful or problematic *drinking*, but not harmful or problem *drinkers*. It may seem like a small difference, but it's not. Labeling people can be pejorative and can get in the way of needed change. Taking an honest look at your drinking can be hard if you think you might have to call yourself "alcoholic." When we ask drinkers to tell us how alcohol has caused problems for them, they usually can give us a long list; yet the very same people, when asked, "Are you a problem drinker?" say "No." Taking a close look at what you are doing does not have to evoke shame or blame. We urge you not to worry about personal labels and consider instead what is actually happening in your life with regard to alcohol.

What to Do?

One reasonable solution, if you're having problems related to alcohol, is to stop drinking altogether. As with smoking, many people choose to refrain from alcohol. Sometimes this is the wisest and even the easiest solution.

ALCOHOL FACTS

In annual surveys of the U.S. population, a "current drinker" is defined as anyone who had at least one drink containing alcohol within the past month. These percentages have changed relatively little over the past two decades. As of the 2010 national survey, these were the percentages:

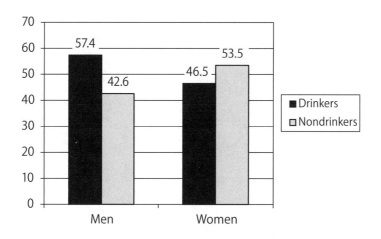

Source: U.S. Substance Abuse and Mental Health Services Administration, Office of Applied Studies, National Survey on Drug Use and Health.

For people whose liver has been damaged by alcohol or disease, further drinking can be life threatening, and abstinence would be the wisest course. Those who have already overcome a drinking problem by becoming totally abstinent are also well advised to stay that way. After all, this is a way to know for sure that alcohol is not going to harm you. About one-third of American adults don't drink at all (see Chapter 4), and almost half drink less often than once a month.

Not everyone who overdrinks, however, chooses to stop drinking altogether. Like moderation, abstinence can be challenging to maintain. Even after treatment with an abstinence goal, an average of three out of four people drink again at some time.[3] Others would simply prefer to continue drinking if they can do so safely. For these and other reasons, people seek to reduce and manage their own drinking without stopping completely. Chapter 2 is designed to help you decide whether this is what you want to do, and Chapter 3 offers some questions that you can answer for yourself from which we can tell you about the likelihood that moderation will work for you. This book was written specifically for people who want to give moderation a try and is designed to help you do five things:

1. Understand how alcohol affects your body and mind, and when your risk of harm becomes significant.
2. Become aware of factors that may be contributing to your overdrinking and the extent to which drinking may be controlling you.
3. Understand what you get out of drinking that may interfere with your successfully cutting down or quitting.
4. Learn what you can do before and while you drink, to prevent overdrinking and related harm.
5. Learn new ways to do for yourself whatever alcohol does for you.

But that's getting ahead of the story.

2

•

Why Change?

Many people who read this book are ambivalent about drinking, and that's quite normal. There are things to like about alcohol and also some not-so-good things. A first step in any change is deciding whether to do it.

As a starting point, we suggest that you make a list of your reasons to continue drinking as you have been and also a list of reasons to cut down (or quit) drinking. Don't just *think* about it—use the blank form on the next page and actually try this.

On the left side of the form, make your list of the arguments to keep on drinking as you have been. This can include things that you like about alcohol or drinking, things that you might miss if you cut back or quit. This is one side of the scales—the reasons *not* to cut down.

On the other side, the right side of the page, make a second list of the less good aspects of drinking for you. Here it might be helpful to look through the questionnaire in Appendix B, which is essentially a list of things that sometimes happen to people in relation to overdrinking. Your list, though, should contain those things that matter to you or to people you care about. If you were to make a good case for cutting down on your drinking, what would the most persuasive reasons be? One person's list is shown on page 13.

What are the things on *your* two lists? Keep in mind that the things you like about alcohol don't have to be positive pleasures. They can be a problem solved or avoided (such as forgetting about worries) or the release of inhibitions (such as getting past shyness). Similarly, your reasons to cut down don't have to be "bad" things to escape but can include positive things that could come from making a change in your drinking. Your list can also contain more than logical reasons. Sometimes drinking is irrational or emotional. List whatever occurs to you.

Weighing the Pros and Cons

Reasons to keep drinking the way I have been	Reasons to cut down or quit

Here is one of several points in this book at which you may feel a bit reluctant or uneasy. That's perfectly natural. Taking an honest look at drinking makes some people want to shut the book, turn away, maybe even have a drink! You decide, of course, how far and how fast to go. We just want to say that if making this list—or doing some other steps later on in this book—makes you uncomfortable, that's really normal. Also, feeling uncomfortable doesn't mean that you have to turn away.

It's perfectly normal to feel uncomfortable about taking an honest look at your drinking.

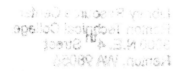

Weighing the Pros and Cons

Reasons to keep drinking the way I have been	Reasons to cut down or quit
Helps me relax and unwind at the end of the day Feel high Forget about my worries Being with my friends I like the taste Too hard to change	I'd feel better in the morning I have trouble remembering things sometimes Good for my health in the long run My work suffers sometimes My family is worried that I drink too much Will help my self-image

Courage, it is said, is not the absence of discomfort, but rather moving ahead in spite of it.

Now, considering the list you've made, as well as any other things that occur to you, how *important* would you say that it is to you to make a change in your drinking? Give yourself a rating, from 0 to 10:

How important is it?

0	1	2	3	4	5	6	7	8	9	10
Not at all important										Extremely important

Chances are that you didn't choose zero as your importance rating. Otherwise you wouldn't be reading this book. So why did you choose the number that you did instead of a lower number or zero? Write down your reasons for choosing this number.

_____

_____

_____

_____

Then give yourself a second rating. How *confident* are you that if you *did* decide to cut down you could reduce your drinking to a moderate level and keep it there?

How confident are you that you could moderate your drinking if you decided to?										
0	1	2	3	4	5	6	7	8	9	10
Not at all confident										Totally confident

And finally, how confident are you that if you did decide to *quit*, you could stop drinking and remain abstinent?

How confident are you that you could quit drinking if you decided to?										
0	1	2	3	4	5	6	7	8	9	10
Not at all confident										Totally confident

The best "how to change" advice is of little use until you yourself decide that it's important and possible to change. Is your importance rating high enough to make it worth the effort? If your importance rating is on the low side (for example, 3 or less), what might cause that number to increase? Some things that people have said that might increase their importance ratings are:

- "If I had a really negative thing happen, like losing my job."
- "If I started drinking in the morning."
- "If I had a blackout."
- "If I thought I was hurting my family."
- "If I was arrested."

How about your confidence? Do you think you could moderate your drinking if you set your mind to it? Perhaps the specific ideas in the chapters that follow will increase your confidence, or at least give you a clearer picture of what is involved. If your confidence is low right now, you might want to come back to this scale after reading the rest of the book and see if your confidence has increased. Do you think you're more likely to succeed, in the long run, by moderating your drinking or by quitting altogether? What's your best guess? People give all kinds of answers here:

- "I'm pretty sure (8) I could quit if I knew I had to, but I'm not so sure (4) about being able to cut down, though I'd like to."
- "I don't think I could quit for the rest of my life (2), and I'm only a little more confident about cutting down (3)."
- "I really think that I can drink in moderation (9)."
- "I've tried before to cut down, so I'm a little discouraged (5), not as sure as I was. Maybe this will help me. If not, I know I can always quit (10)."

Outcomes of This Program

Whatever you choose to do, think of it as an experiment. Try out this new way of being and see how it feels, how it works for you. Chances are your own experience will be like one of the following five patterns:

Whatever you choose to do, think of it as an experiment.

1. **Stable moderation**. Some people have found that moderation works well for them and that once they've cut down it's no longer a struggle. They can take a drink or leave it. Alcohol becomes unimportant to them. They don't feel like "controlled" drinkers. Some days they don't drink at all. At other times they have a drink or two without wanting or needing more. Their drinking poses no real problems for them or others, and they are comfortable with moderation.

2. **Pretty good moderation**. Like the Stable Moderation group, these people also cut way back on their drinking. They still had some days when they drank too much, and now and then they still had problems related to their drinking, but nothing like before.

3. **White-knuckle moderation**. Others gradually tapered their drinking but found that it was a continual struggle to keep it under control. They felt as though they were walking a tightrope from which they might fall at any time. They could do it, but it was an awful lot of work, and it didn't seem to get any easier over time. They drank less but still wanted more. In the long run, these people usually decided it wasn't worth the effort, and they quit drinking altogether. If down the line they did happen to have a drink, they usually didn't go all out. Instead, they tended to go right back to being nondrinkers within a day or two.

4. **Pointless moderation**. Still others succeeded in moderating their drinking and may not have experienced it as a struggle to stay there. They wondered, however, what the point was in drinking so little. Previously they drank to get drunk, and having achieved moderation, they found that alcohol had lost its meaning. As with the stable moderation group, alcohol no longer mattered to them, but like the white-knuckle moderation group, they tended to quit drinking altogether. They tapered to the point at which alcohol no longer mattered, and then they quit. Again, if down the line they did happen to have a drink, they tended to go right back to abstaining within a few days. It just reminded them of the pointlessness of drinking.

5. **Nice try moderation**. Then there was a group composed of those who really tried to moderate their drinking but didn't have much success with it. They cut back some and had days or weeks of moderation, but like a sponge that had been compressed, their drinking tended to pop right back to its original shape. The experience of having given it a good but unsuccessful try, even with the best self-management methods available, helped them let go of the idea of controlling their drinking, and they chose to abstain rather than allow alcohol to continue harming them and others.

All five of these are happy outcomes. Chances are that if you're reading this book, you're hoping to wind up with stable moderation, or at least with pretty good moderation. People in groups 3, 4, and 5 all tend to wind up abstaining, but for different reasons. Those in group 3 quit because it's too hard to maintain moderation. Those in group 4 simply don't care for moderation; they see no point in it. Those in group 5 tried moderation but found they couldn't do it.

It is disturbingly common for authors of self-help books to make highly optimistic claims, to give pump-you-up promises about how successful you're going to be if you just follow their advice. We would love to paint a rosy picture for you, but most of all we want to give you an honest picture of what you might expect, based on our research following participants in our program over periods of 3 to 8 years afterward.[4] To keep ourselves honest, we included in our follow-up team a psychiatric colleague who was highly skeptical about helping people moderate their drinking. Our conclusions were conservative, based on consensus agreement with our skeptical colleague about the outcomes our participants had experienced. The findings regarding stable moderation were neither as high as we had expected nor as low as our consultant had predicted. Over 12 months prior to follow-up:

- One in seven (15%) had maintained stable moderation throughout the year (staying under three drinks per day and averaging 10 standard drinks per week) without any alcohol-related problems or signs of alcohol dependence.
- Another 23% had "pretty good moderation," reducing their drinking by two-thirds or more (averaging about 14 drinks per week), but continued to experience some alcohol-related problems, at least occasionally.
- A further one in four (24%) had been totally abstinent for at least a year. These would be people who experienced moderation as too difficult, pointless, or unattainable.
- And that left 37% who were still drinking heavily or harmfully 1 year later.

What if you could predict which group you'll be in? Chapter 3 may help you estimate in advance how likely you are to maintain moderate and problem-free drinking. Size up your options, using the information in the next two chapters, and then figure out what you want to do. If you decide to give moderation a try, give it a good one. If you try this program and find yourself among those who continue to drink excessively despite your best efforts, you can always decide to quit, and could seek help in doing so. As we emphasized before, there are many different ways to get past problematic drinking, [5,6] and if one doesn't work for you, it only means that *this one* didn't work for you. Try something else. Part V of this book is particularly for people in this last group who have difficulty moderating and need some additional help to decide on, reach, and maintain abstinence.

A trap to avoid is expecting perfection. Most people don't change

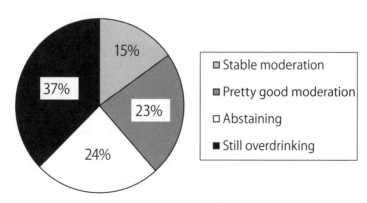

One-year outcomes from this program.

> *Personal Reflection*
>
> In college during the 1960s I decided not to drink. I was already in the habit of passing on the joints smoked at parties in my dorm, and when I realized that alcohol came with even greater risks, I decided there was no point in drinking either. At first I thought that I had to explain why I didn't drink at each social event. Then I decided it was unnecessary, especially when it became clear that my explanations were often interpreted as criticisms of those who did drink. That wasn't my intent, so I stopped explaining. Soon I realized most people didn't even notice I wasn't drinking anything alcoholic anyway!
>
> The decision not to drink is a personal one, and it can sometimes be easier to follow through on your decision when you don't try to justify it.
>
> —RFM

completely or all at once. New Year's resolutions often fail because once the new rule has been broken, the person gives up. People who are trying to quit drinking altogether can fall into this trap: having taken one drink (or one too many), they say "Now I've done it! I'm off my program. I've blown my goal. All that progress is lost." Studying more than 8,000 people who had received treatment for alcohol problems,[7] we first removed all those who had been completely abstinent for 1 year (24%). Some might regard the remaining 76% as treatment "failures" because they had not stopped drinking completely. Yet on average these people had reduced their drinking by 87% (from 77 to 10 drinks per week, on average!), and their alcohol-related problems had diminished by 60%. Don't stop trying because you're not perfect.

Avoid the trap of expecting perfection.

A Self-Management Toolbox

People sometimes talk about willpower, as if simply setting your mind to abstain or drink moderately should be enough. Then, when their intention falters and they drink more than planned, they feel weak-willed or a failure. Perhaps you have already tried once or more to quit or cut down on sheer willpower and found it difficult. Maybe others have told you—or you have told yourself—that you ought to be able to just make up your mind and do it.

We recommend a different approach that involves a set of tools to help you reach your goals. You might think of these as self-help or self-management skills. This book is a box of such tools—methods that other people have found useful in managing their own behavior (in this case, drinking). Self-management has to do not only with willing or wanting, but also with doing. The subsequent sections of this book describe three broad sets of self-management tools that you can use. When we asked people who succeeded in using this book how they did it, they usually told us they chose a small set of tools that seemed as if they would work for them and then *put them into practice*. Reading about tools doesn't get the job done; it's choosing the right tools and using them that makes change happen.

- **When you drink.** One necessary step toward moderation is to change what you do *while* you are drinking—to change the way you drink. Because most problems with alcohol have to do with overdrinking, one thing you can do is to change your *rate* of drinking. That can be more challenging than it sounds, because drinking rapidly becomes a habit that takes on a life of its own. Perhaps you're not consciously aware of your rate of drinking; you just do it. Part II of this book will offer you some systematic ways to consciously slow down your drinking.
- **Before you drink.** A second way of gaining greater self-control is to understand what triggers your drinking. This involves examining the situations in which you drink and the things that happen just before you drink. Some people drink more when they are with certain people or on certain days of the week or at certain times of day. Others overdrink when they are feeling certain ways: stressed, down, angry, or celebrative. Part III of this book will teach you ways to plan ahead and moderate your drinking by understanding and changing the things that trigger it.
- **Instead of drinking.** Many people drink (and overdrink) because of the effects that alcohol has on them. Some of these effects are obvious (such as intoxication), but others are more subtle. Part IV of this book will help you explore the positive effects that you anticipate from drinking. If you understand what you hope to happen when you use alcohol, you may be able to find alternative ways of accomplishing the same thing. Suppose, for example, that you use alcohol to relax, to get to sleep, or to feel better. These are desirable states, but if alcohol is the *only* way you have to get there, you're stuck. Part IV can be useful whether your chosen goal is moderation or abstinence. Alternatives give you freedom of choice about drinking and form a third road to self-control.

3

•

Is Moderation for You?

No one approach is good for everyone. A diet that can help one person lose weight safely may be ineffective or hazardous for another. Over-the-counter or prescription medications can be beneficial, but if used improperly they can be harmful or even fatal. Similarly, there are now many different approaches for overcoming problems with alcohol, and the method described in this book is only one alternative. The good news is that there is a menu of effective alternatives from which to choose. This chapter is designed to help you determine whether the approach described in this book is likely to work for you, based on currently available research.

Research on Moderation

One question to consider is: What kind of person seems to be most successful in learning and maintaining moderate drinking? A number of studies have examined this question, and the answer has been reasonably consistent: people who take action while their problems with and dependence on alcohol are *less severe* have the easiest time of it. In general, the people who are more likely to achieve and maintain moderation:

- Have had enough problems with alcohol to be concerned about their drinking, but it has not yet caused *major* life disruption.
- Recognize that they have problems with drinking but do not regard themselves as alcoholic (although they may wonder at times).
- Have less family history of severe alcohol problems and dependence.
- Have had alcohol-related problems for less than 10 years.
- Have not been physically addicted to alcohol (that is, can go for a

20

week or two without taking alcohol or tranquilizers and not have unpleasant physical symptoms of withdrawal).

This includes a broad range of people. Here are some examples:

- **Joseph.** This middle-aged man had quit for 2 months because his family was very concerned about how much he had been drinking. Although he had been drinking quite a bit, he felt no discomfort (withdrawal) when he stopped abruptly. He had a good job and hadn't really experienced significant troubles related to drinking, except at home. "I know I'm going to drink again," he said. "When I do, I'd like to keep it moderate and make sure I don't overdo it."
- **Ruth.** Ruth was shocked to have been arrested for drunk driving after a few beers. Her name and picture appeared in the newspaper, and she was embarrassed. "I didn't even feel intoxicated," she said. "I felt absolutely fine, but when they tested me I was at twice the legal limit. I don't ever want to go through that again."
- **C. J.** "I'm not sure what to do," this 20-something man told us. "I know I'm drinking way too much for my own good. I thought I'd grow out of it after college, but it didn't happen, and I wind up doing things and taking chances I'd never take if I was sober. But I just can't see myself abstaining for the rest of my life!"
- **Chris.** "Now that I'm married, I guess I need to settle down some," this newlywed told us. "I used to go down to Mexico with friends and have a great time. I love to party. Eventually we'll have kids, though, and then I'll have to do things differently, but I'm just not quite ready to give up the good times."
- **Fran.** Before retiring, Fran never really drank all that much. Suddenly there was all this leisure time. "My work was my whole life, and I didn't do much else. Now that I'm home alone, I pass the time sipping wine until I fall asleep. When the doctor asked me how much I was drinking, and I told her, she said I should come talk to you."

There are also some important practical considerations. We do not recommend even moderate alcohol consumption:

- If you are pregnant or might become pregnant, because alcohol is dangerous to an unborn child from the day of conception, and there is no known safe level of drinking during pregnancy.

- If you have a medical condition (such as liver disease or a stomach ulcer) that could be made worse by any drinking. Your physician should evaluate this. If you have not had a thorough physical examination recently, we strongly recommend that you do so before starting this program.
- If you tend to lose control of your behavior (for example, tend to become aggressive or violent) when you drink even small amounts of alcohol.
- If you drive with alcohol in your system. Even one incident of driving under the influence could end your life or someone else's life.
- If you are taking tranquilizers, sedatives, sleeping pills, or any other medication that is dangerous when combined with alcohol. Ask your pharmacist!
- Finally, we add the practical point that if you have been refraining from alcohol successfully for a year or more, we recommend that you stick with abstinence.

Two Self-Evaluations

From our follow-up studies with people who have tried this self-control approach (either with a counselor or via this book), we have been able to predict who will do well with moderation. We gave these two widely

You can estimate ahead of time how likely you are to succeed with moderation.

used questionnaires to people entering our self-control training program. You can match your own answers to how they responded and determine your scores on these two scales. Then, from your scores, we can give you an estimate of your own chances of succeeding with moderation versus abstinence, based on the outcomes for people previously trying this approach.

The Michigan Alcoholism Screening Test

The first questionnaire consists of two dozen questions and is known as the Michigan Alcoholism Screening Test (MAST).[8] It's a broad set of questions, designed to screen for (but not diagnose) problems related to alcohol. (*Screening* is the process of checking for the possibility of a problem, whereas *diagnosis* is the confirmation of a problem.) Answer the questions honestly for yourself by circling either Yes or No for each item.

The MAST

1. Do you feel you are a normal drinker?	No 2	Yes 0
2. Have you ever awakened the morning after some drinking the night before and found that you could not remember a part of the evening before?	No 0	Yes 2
3. Does any member of your family (wife, husband, parents, etc.) ever worry or complain about your drinking?	No 0	Yes 1
4. Can you stop drinking without a struggle after one or two drinks?	No 2	Yes 0
5. Do you ever feel bad about your drinking?	No 0	Yes 1
6. Do friends or relatives think you are a normal drinker?	No 1	Yes 0
7. Are you always able to stop drinking when you want to?	No 2	Yes 0
8. Have you ever attended a meeting of Alcoholics Anonymous (AA)?	No 0	Yes 5
9. Have you gotten into fights when drinking?	No 0	Yes 1
10. Has drinking ever created problems with you and your spouse (husband/wife)?	No 0	Yes 2
11. Has your spouse (or other family member) ever gone to anyone for help about your drinking?	No 0	Yes 2
12. Have you ever lost friends or lovers because of your drinking?	No 0	Yes 2
13. Have you ever gotten into trouble at work because of drinking?	No 0	Yes 2
14. Have you ever lost a job because of drinking?	No 0	Yes 2
15. Have you ever neglected your obligations, your family, or your work for two or more days in a row because you were drinking?	No 0	Yes 2
16. Do you ever drink before noon?	No 0	Yes 1

(cont.)

	No	Yes
17. Have you ever been told you have liver trouble?	No 0	Yes 2
18. After heavy drinking, have you ever had severe shaking or heard voices or seen things that weren't there?	No 0	Yes 2
19. Have you ever gone to anyone for help about your drinking?	No 0	Yes 5
20. Have you ever been in a hospital because of drinking?	No 0	Yes 5
21. Have you ever been a patient in a psychiatric hospital or on a psychiatric ward of a general hospital?	No 0	Yes 2
22. Have you ever been seen at a psychiatric or mental health clinic, or gone to a doctor, social worker, or clergy for help with an emotional problem?	No 0	Yes 2
23. Have you ever been arrested, even for a few hours, because of drunk behavior? (other than driving)	No 0	Yes 2
24. Have you ever been arrested for drunk driving or driving after drinking?	No 0	Yes 2

Source: Selzer, M. L. (1971). The Michigan Alcohol Screening Test: The quest for a new diagnostic instrument. *American Journal of Psychiatry, 127*(12), 1653–1658. Copyright 1971 by the American Psychiatric Association; *http://ajp.psychiatryonline.org.* Reprinted by permission.

Now total up your score for all the answers you circled. For example, if you answered "No" to the first question, you would give yourself 2 points, but if you answered "Yes," you would add zero points to your score for question #1. Your score is the total of points for all the answers you circled.

The Alcohol Dependence Scale

The second questionnaire, the Alcohol Dependence Scale (ADS)[9] (on pp. 25–27), was designed specifically to evaluate a person's level of dependence on alcohol. "Dependence" here does not refer just to physical addiction. *Alcohol dependence* is a pattern in which one's life becomes increasingly centered around and reliant upon drinking. Again, answer the questions honestly for yourself by putting a check mark in one box for each item. Do it now.

The Alcohol Dependence Scale

1. How much did you drink the last time you drank?	____ Enough to get high or less 0	____ Enough to get drunk 1	____ Enough to pass out 2
2. Do you often have hangovers on Sunday or Monday mornings?	____ No 0		____ Yes 1
3. Have you had the "shakes" when sobering up (hands tremble, shake inside)?	____ No 0	____ Sometimes 1	____ Almost every time I drink 2
4. Do you get physically sick (e.g., vomit, stomach cramps) as a result of drinking?	____ No 0	____ Sometimes 1	____ Almost every time I drink 2
5. Have you had the "DTs" (delirium tremens)—that is, seen, felt, or heard things not really there; felt very anxious, restless, and overexcited?	____ No 0	____ Once 1	____ Several times 2
6. When you drink, do you stumble about, stagger, and weave?	____ No 0	____ Sometimes 1	____ Often 2
7. As a result of drinking, have you felt overly hot and sweaty (feverish)?	____ No 0	____ Once 1	____ Several times 2
8. As a result of drinking, have you seen things that were not really there?	____ No 0	____ Once 1	____ Several times 2
9. Do you panic because you fear you may not have a drink when you need it?	____ No 0		____ Yes 1
10. Have you had blackouts ("loss of memory" without passing out) as a result of drinking?	____ No 0 ____ Some-times 1	____ Often 2	____ Almost every time I drink 3
11. Do you carry a bottle with you or keep one close at hand?	____ No 0	____ Some of the time 1	____ Most of the time 2

(cont.)

12. After a period of abstinence (not drinking), do you end up drinking heavily again?	____ No 0	____ Sometimes 1	____ Almost every time 2
13. In the past 12 months, have you passed out as a result of drinking?	____ No 0	____ Once 1	____ More than once 2
14. Have you had a convulsion (fit) following a period of drinking?	____ No 0	____ Once 1	____ Several times 2
15. Do you drink throughout the day?	____ No 0	____ Yes 1	
16. After drinking heavily, has your thinking been fuzzy or unclear?	____ No 0	____ Yes, but only for a few hours 1	____ Yes, for one or two days 2 ____ Yes, for many days 3
17. As a result of drinking, have you felt your heart beating rapidly?	____ No 0	____ Once 1	____ Several times 2
18. Do you almost constantly think about drinking and alcohol?	____ No 0	____ Yes 1	
19. As a result of drinking, have you heard "things" that were not really there?	____ No 0	____ Once 1	____ Several times 2
20. Have you had weird and frightening sensations when drinking?	____ No 0	____ Once or twice 1	____ Often 2
21. As a result of drinking, have you "felt things" crawling on you that were not really there (e.g., bugs, spiders)?	____ No 0	____ Once 1	____ Several times 2
22. With respect to blackouts (loss of memory):	____ Have never had a blackout 0	____ Have had blackouts that last less than an hour 1	____ Have had blackouts that last for several hours 2 ____ Have had blackouts that last for a day or more 3
23. Have you tried to cut down on your drinking and failed?	____ No 0	____ Yes 1	

| 24. Do you gulp drinks (drink quickly)? | ____ No 0 | ____ Yes 1 |
| 25. After taking one or two drinks, can you usually stop? | ____ No 1 | ____ Yes 0 |

Source: Horn, J., Skinner, H. A., Wanberg, K., & Foster, F. M. (1984). *The Alcohol Dependence Scale (ADS).* Toronto, Ontario, Canada: Centre for Addiction and Mental Health. Copyright 1984 by the Centre for Addiction and Mental Health and Harvey A. Skinner. Reprinted by permission.

Once you have finished the ADS, total up your score. For each one of the 25 items, add the number of points shown in the lower right-hand corner of the box you checked. For example, if you answered "No" to question #3, do not add any points to your score, but if you answered "Sometimes," then add 1 point to your score, and if you answered "Almost every time I drink," add 2 points to your score. Your total score is the sum of all of your points for the 25 items.

What Do Your Scores Tell You?

The MAST is a reasonably good measure of the extent of problems related to drinking. According to the scale's author, a score of 5 or higher indicates possible reason for concern. People seeking professional treatment for problems with drinking often score 20 or higher on the MAST, though there is wide variation.

The ADS, on the other hand, indicates the extent to which you have developed a behavioral pattern of dependence on alcohol. Again, most people entering treatment for alcohol problems score above 20 on this scale, but with wide variation. The scale's authors suggested the following interpretation[10]:

Score range	Meaning
1–13	Low level of alcohol dependence
14–21	Moderate level of alcohol dependence
22–30	Substantial level of alcohol dependence
31–47	Severe level of alcohol dependence

We gave the same two questionnaires to people who were beginning the self-control program described in this book. Then we followed them over a period of up to 8 years and determined who had maintained moderate drinking and who had quit drinking altogether. These two groups (abstainers and moderate drinkers) had scored very differently on both questionnaires. Hoping that this information will be helpful in your own decision making, we offer the summary in the boxes on page 29. Of course, as in all treatment studies, some participants (about one-third) continued to drink heavily during the period of follow-up.

One more finding from our research is noteworthy here. In our studies, people were randomly assigned to work on their own by following instructions in this self-help book or to receive the same program by meeting weekly with a counselor for between 6 and 18 weeks. We found that those using this book on a self-help basis were just as successful as those working with a counselor. Their outcomes were the same on average as those reported above.

Now What?

You've reached a choice point. Based on your reasons for making a change in your drinking (Chapter 2) and what you've learned here about your likelihood of succeeding with moderation versus abstinence, what are you going to do? If you decide that abstinence is best and you want some help in quitting, a number of good treatment approaches and other resources are available (see Chapter 30). You may also find useful the material in Part IV of this book ("Instead of Drinking"), which describes alcohol-free ways to accomplish what people sometimes want or hope that drinking will do for them. If, on the other hand, you decide you want to try to achieve moderation, read on. The methods described in this book are the best that we have to offer you for moderating your drinking. If you think you can maintain moderate drinking, give it a good effort.[11]

If the methods we describe work for you, you've learned what you wanted to know. And if, by chance, you find that moderation doesn't work for you, what you learn will still be useful in helping you plan how to proceed.

Here are the decisions made by some of the people we met earlier:

Despite his rather heavy drinking, Joseph scored in the medium range on the MAST and the low range of the ADS. He stayed away from alcohol for 2 months but knew that he did not want to remain abstinent and decided to go ahead with a moderation program.

MAST SCORES AND MODERATION

People who scored in this range on the MAST . . .		Showed these outcomes with regard to abstinence and moderation
Low	0–10	These people were the most likely to moderate their drinking with few or no problems. They were less likely to stop drinking altogether, although one in six did ultimately decide to quit.
Medium	11–18	People in this group were about equally likely to abstain or to attain moderate and problem-free drinking. Others in this group reduced their drinking substantially but continued to experience some problems.
High	19–28	This group was most likely to become completely abstinent. Only one in 12 maintained moderate and problem-free drinking. Most who overcame their drinking problems did so by stopping completely.
Very high	29 or higher	These people had the most difficulty. Everyone in this group who overcame his or her drinking problems did so by abstaining. In our studies, no one with a score this high has ever succeeded in maintaining problem-free moderation.

ADS SCORES AND MODERATION

People who scored in this range on the ADS . . .		Showed these outcomes with regard to abstinence and moderation
Low	0–14	These people were the most likely to moderate their drinking with few or no problems. They were less likely to stop drinking altogether, although one in 12 did ultimately decide to quit.
Medium	15–20	People in this group were about equally likely to abstain or to attain moderate and problem-free drinking. Others reduced their drinking substantially but continued to experience some problems.
High	21–27	People in this group were about twice as likely to abstain as to maintain problem-free moderation. Only one in five maintained moderate and problem-free drinking.
Very high	28 or higher	Everyone in this group who overcame his or her drinking problems did so by abstaining. In our studies, no one with a score this high ever succeeded in maintaining problem-free moderation.

Just 2 years out of college, C. J. was stunned by the test results, scoring in the very high range on the MAST and the high range on the ADS. C. J.'s father had had severe problems with alcohol and had died in his 50s from pancreatic cancer. It was a tough pill to swallow, but considering the odds, C. J. decided it would be best to stay away from alcohol altogether. The challenge, of course, was how to have friends, fun, and a rewarding life when alcohol had become so central. We worked with C. J. to make the shift, using some of the methods described in Part IV.

Fran scored between Joseph and C. J. on these two questionnaires: high on the MAST and medium on the ADS. The odds favored abstinence over moderation, but Fran had already tried several times to stop drinking altogether, without success. The moderation program offered a new option, and Fran definitely wanted to give it a try.

Personal Reflection: Wanting versus Choosing

I have Type 2 diabetes, and sometimes people ask me, "Can you have dessert?" Soon after my diagnosis I was struggling with the idea that "I can't have sweets." I wanted to rebel against the idea that "I can't." Then it hit me that I *can* have sweets (I am certainly able to), and sometimes I would *like* to, but I *choose* not to in the interest of my health. I found this way of thinking about it to be liberating. It is an antidote for thinking I'm being confined or deprived and feeling sorry for myself. There is no one else deciding this for me. I choose to be careful about what I eat because I want to stay healthy.

I find that the same often applies to drinking. Thinking "I can't drink" does work for some people, but others want to rebel against it. A fellow I was working with once seemed to have decided that he would quit drinking to protect his family. "So is that what you want to do?" I asked. "No," he said. "It's not what I *want* to do; it's what I'm *going* to do because it's the right thing." You don't even have to *want* to make a change to do it!

—WRM

Part II

•

When You Drink

If you've read this far, we assume you're ready to get down to business, or at least to consider how you might go about moderating your drinking. The chapters in Part II offer you practical methods for cutting down on drinking. This is only one part of the picture, of course. Later sections address things to do before you drink (Part III) and instead of drinking (Part IV). Here the focus is on changing your pattern of drinking.

Some people are reasonably steady drinkers. They consume about the same amount of alcohol on most days. They may not experience their drinking as being out of control. It's just that the amount they drink is too high. The more dependent they've become on alcohol, the more challenging it is to reduce their drinking to a moderate and problem-free level.

Other people overdo it periodically. They drink too much in too short a time and suffer the consequences. Their risk has to do not so much with the amount they drink every day but with how much they drink at some times and in certain situations. In between, they may drink moderately or not at all. Then, of course, there are those who both overdrink on a daily basis and have heavier episodes of drinking.

Whatever your own pattern, this section outlines ways in which you can systematically work on moderating your drinking. The goal is to reduce your use below levels that produce harm and place you or others at risk.

An Experiment in Freedom

Human beings are quite susceptible to habit—to developing behavior patterns that become more or less automatic. Overdrinking is like that, a habit that proceeds without your thinking very much about it. Much of Part II is about changing an established habit and replacing it with a new automatic pattern of moderation. One way to make such a transition is to consciously break the old habit before establishing a new one.

Although it may seem odd, one good way to get a head start on moderating your drinking is to take a temporary vacation from alcohol. Some people have found it very helpful, before beginning this program, to try a period of 2 weeks without alcohol. There are several good reasons to do this:

1. It breaks the prior habits of drinking and gives you a head start on learning new ones.
2. It is a surefire way, provided you don't take any substitute drugs such as tranquilizers or sedatives, to establish that you are not *physically* addicted to alcohol (see the next section).
3. It demonstrates that you can do without alcohol for a period of time.
4. It helps you discover how other parts of your life are intertwined with drinking, to identify ways in which you may be *psychologically* dependent on alcohol.
5. Last but not least, you may find that you like abstaining, and choose to continue.

In a way, this is an experiment in freedom, to explore how free you are to manage your own drinking.

Many people beginning this program of self-control have been willing to try this vacation from alcohol.[12] Truly moderate drinking, after all, does involve increasing one's days and hours of abstinence. If you find yourself resisting the idea of giving up alcohol even for 2 weeks, then this experiment in freedom may be all the *more* important for you.

The choice, of course, is yours to make. This is not a *necessary* first step. If you choose not to begin with a 2-week period of nondrinking, you can still make use of all the methods that follow. We do, however, recommend it as an experiment in freedom.

Physical Addiction to Alcohol

Alcohol is a drug capable of creating strong physical addiction. When you consume large quantities of alcohol over a period of time, your body may come to rely on the presence of alcohol to function normally. If the alcohol supply is then suddenly decreased or cut off completely, the body may respond negatively in various ways for a few days. This process is termed *abstinence syndrome*, and the body's negative reactions are known as *withdrawal symptoms*. People differ greatly with regard to addiction and withdrawal. Some become physically dependent on alcohol rather quickly. Others drink for many years without showing major signs of alcohol withdrawal when they quit.

At any rate, you should be prepared for the possibility that your body will react negatively when you begin to reduce your drinking. If physical dependence is strong, withdrawal from alcohol can be far more dangerous than withdrawal from heroin.

Usually the body's protest is mild if alcohol consumption is reduced gradually, but you may experience some withdrawal symptoms. These can range from a headache, vague feelings of tension, or "the shakes," to severe reactions such as hallucinations or convulsions. If you experience discomfort as you begin to decrease your drinking, you should consult your doctor immediately. A physician is the best person to judge the seriousness of withdrawal symptoms and to see you safely through them. In general, your risk of significant withdrawal symptoms is higher if:

- You drink large quantities of alcohol on a daily basis.
- It has been a long time since you went for even a few days without any alcohol (or other drugs, such as antianxiety medications, that substitute for alcohol).
- In the past, when you've stopped drinking for a day or more, your body reacted negatively.

With proper medical supervision, withdrawal from alcohol is safe and relatively painless. When in doubt, see your personal physician.

4

●

Getting Started

Setting Limits

An important first step in making any intentional change is to have a clear goal in mind. Setting clear limits for yourself is perhaps the simplest strategy for moderating your drinking, and it's often the first thing that people try.

What should your limits be? That's up to you, of course, but here is some information to help you to decide.

What Is a "Drink"?

What people mean by a "drink" varies widely. For one woman we treated, a drink was an 8-ounce (250-ml) glass filled almost to the rim with gin, topped off with a touch of vermouth. When she said that she had had only two drinks, she meant something different from the man who said he drank two cans of beer.

So we need a common working definition of what constitutes a drink. Fortunately, all alcohol beverages contain the same kind of alcohol, known as ethanol or ethyl alcohol. This allows all drinks to be converted into a standard drink unit, the size of which varies across countries.[13]

In the United States we have defined *one standard drink* as the amount of any beverage that contains ½ ounce (15 ml) of pure ethyl alcohol, which corresponds reasonably well to some common servings of alcohol beverages. One-half ounce is the amount of alcohol contained in each of the following:

A 10-ounce (300-ml) glass of beer (5% alcohol)
A 12-ounce (350-ml) can of light beer (4.2% alcohol)

A 4-ounce (125-ml) glass of table wine (12% alcohol)

A 2½-ounce (75-ml) glass of fortified wine (20% alcohol) such as sherry, port, or brandy

A 1¼-ounce (35-ml) shot (slight overpour) of 80-proof liquor (40% alcohol)

A 1-ounce (30-ml) shot of 100-proof liquor (50% alcohol)

Each of these drinks contains about the *same amount (½ ounce) of the same kind* of alcohol. All of the tables and discussion in this book are based on this standard drink unit.

If you like math, it's simple enough to calculate exactly how much ethyl alcohol you are consuming. (If you don't enjoy math, just skip this paragraph.) Multiply the number of ounces of beverage by the proportion of alcohol that it contains. If you know the U.S. "proof" of a beverage, divide it in half to get the percentage of alcohol (86 proof = 43%). For example:

Six pack of beer	72 ounces × .05	=	3.6 ounces of alcohol or 7.2 drinks
Fifth of wine	25.6 ounces × .12	=	3.07 ounces of alcohol or 6.1 drinks
Pint of sherry	16 ounces × .20	=	3.2 ounces of alcohol or 6.4 drinks
Pint of 86 proof	16 ounces × .43	=	6.88 ounces of alcohol or 13.8 drinks

Notice that the number of standard drinks is just twice the number of ounces of alcohol. That simplicity is another good reason for using half an ounce of alcohol as the standard drink unit. One ounce of pure alcohol = two standard drinks.

Recommended Daily Limits to Avoid Harmful Drinking

Various medical and scientific organizations have issued guidelines for safe drinking, usually in the form of a recommended maximum number of drinks per day. As discussed in Chapter 1, the guideline for moderate drinking from the federal agency that funds most U.S. scientific research on alcohol (*www.niaaa.nih.gov*) is that women should have no more than one standard drink per day on average (seven per week), and for men the daily average should be no more than two standard drinks (14 per week). As drinking rises above these limits, so does the risk of problems, illnesses, and all-cause mortality. Most health organizations also recommend not drinking alcohol every day and having some alcohol-free days. Why the sex difference in these guidelines? First of all, men tend to be physically larger than women, and body weight (as you will see later in this chapter) strongly affects the impact of alcohol. Second, men metabolize alcohol more rapidly in the stomach, before it reaches the bloodstream. For this reason, even if a man and a woman of the same body weight drink exactly the same amount of alcohol, the woman is likely to have a significantly higher blood alcohol level and thus be more intoxicated.

If a man and a woman of the same body weight drink exactly the same amount of alcohol, the woman will have a significantly higher blood alcohol level.

The National Average

Another standard for comparison is to ask how much the average person drinks. Before you read any further, make a guess: How many standard drinks (as defined above) would you say the average American man or woman consumes in a typical week?

If you start with the total amount of alcohol apparently consumed in the United States and divide by the number of people over the age of 18, the average person consumes about 2.3 gallons (9 liters) of pure ethyl alcohol per year. This figure—total alcohol consumption—has been gradually decreasing in the United States since the early 1980s. In the 1970s, it was closer to 4 gallons (15 liters) per person per year. The current average of just over 2 gallons (8 liters) comes out to five or six standard drinks per person per week.

However, not everyone drinks alcohol, and the percentage of abstainers in the United States has been increasing gradually. Including abstainers and people who drink only occasionally (less than one drink per week on average), 51% of men and 71% of women drink no alcohol at all in a typical week (see the bar graph on page 38). If the total amount of alcohol consumed is divided by the number of drinkers, then the average is more like 10 standard drinks per week per drinker.

Averages can be misleading, however, because a relatively small proportion of drinkers account for a large amount of the alcohol drunk, and most people consume far less than this "average." In fact, only 18% of men

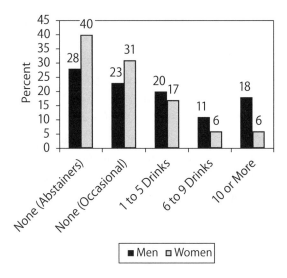

Average number of drinks per week for American men and women.

and 6% of women in the United States *actually* have more than 10 drinks per week on average. It has been estimated that about 80% of all alcoholic beverages are consumed by 20% of the drinkers.

Another way to look at averages, then, is to ask: What percentage of adults in the United States drink as much as I do? This tells you where you stand relative to other people.

So, using the standard drink unit, total up the approximate number of drinks you've been consuming in a typical week. (Be honest with yourself! No one else is looking.) In your average week of drinking:

About how many glasses or cans of beer do you have?   ____
About how many 4-ounce (125-ml) glasses of wine do you have? ____
About how many ½ ounces (15 ml) of liquor do you have?   ____
About how many alcohol drinks of other kinds do you have?   ____
Total drinks per week: ____

Now, in the table on the facing page, find the number of drinks that most closely matches your approximate weekly drinking. The percentage next to it will tell you how many U.S. adults (men or women) out of 100 drink as much as or more than you do. For example, if you look down the page to find how many drink 20 or more drinks per week, you will see that only nine out of 100 adult men and only one out of 100 women drink this much or more.

HOW MANY ADULTS DRINK THAT MUCH OR MORE?

	Men	Women
Abstainers	28%	40%
Occasional drinkers (<1 drink per week)	23%	31%
Percentage of adults who drink less than 1 drink per week (combining the two groups above)	51%	71%
Number of drinks per week: at least . . .		
1	49%	29%
2	40%	21%
3	36%	19%
4	32%	15%
5	29%	12%
6	27%	11%
7	24%	9%
8	21%	7%
9	19%	7%
10	18%	6%
11	17%	5%
12	15%	4%
13	14%	4%
14	13%	3%
15	12%	3%
16–17	11%	2%
18–19	10%	2%
20–21	9%	1%
22–26	8%	1%
27–30	6%	1%
31–36	5%	1%
37–42	4%	< 1%
43–59	3%	< 1%
60–69	2%	< 1%
70 or more	1%	< 1%

Source: Data are from the 2010 National Alcohol Survey (NAS) of 7,969 individuals, residing in 50 states and Washington, DC. The 2010 NAS involved a dual-frame landline household telephone survey augmented by a cell phone sample. The survey included oversamples of African American and Hispanic respondents and also oversampled low-population states. Results are weighted to the 2010 census so as to be representative of the U.S. adult population ages 18 and older. The 2010 NAS was conducted for the National Alcohol Research Center, Alcohol Research Group, Public Health Institute, Emeryville, California, under Center Grant P50-AA05595 (Thomas K. Greenfield, PI) from the National Institute on Alcohol Abuse and Alcoholism (NIAAA). The authors thank Dr. Greenfield and Mr. Yu Ye for their assistance in running this special analysis of the 2010 household data.

A Regular Limit

Now, before it gets any more complicated, consider what you would set as your regular daily limit—the maximum number of drinks that you choose to have per day and per week. (We'll consider special occasions a little later.) Take into account both the recommended daily limits discussed previously and the national drinking data. Based on what you know so far, what might you set as your goal as a limit for:

Number of standard drinks per day? _____
Number of standard drinks per week? _____

Blood Alcohol Concentration (BAC)

Up to this point we've been talking about averages. When it comes to the effects of alcohol on behavior and the body, however, what really counts is how much alcohol is in the blood. It is alcohol in the bloodstream that affects the brain and organs.

The amount of alcohol in the bloodstream is known as the *blood alcohol concentration*, or BAC. The BAC is usually recorded in milligrams of alcohol per 100 milliliters of blood (or milligrams per centum, abbreviated mg%). In the popular press, BAC is often shown as a decimal (such as 0.08 or 0.15), which is just mg% divided by 1,000 (moving the decimal point three places to the left, or g%). We prefer mg%, both because whole numbers can be less confusing than decimals and because BAC is not really a percentage. (Technically, it is a ratio of weight to volume.) Thus from here on in this book we will use the mg% unit whenever we discuss BAC. If you want to convert it into the popular decimal form, however, just move the decimal three places to the left.

A reasonably accurate estimate of one's BAC can be obtained from a breath sample. This is why highway patrols take breath samples to

---

WHAT WOULD YOU GUESS?

Does alcohol generally make one's mood better or worse? _____

The answer is in the "Alcohol Facts" box on page 42.

determine the degree of intoxication of drivers. As you'll see shortly, you can also estimate your BAC at any time if you know a few simple facts. This

Heavier drinkers have a harder time feeling how intoxicated they really are.

is particularly useful because research shows that heavier drinkers often have trouble judging their own level of intoxication just from internal body cues.[14] That is, heavier drinkers have a harder time *feeling* how intoxicated they really are.

Effects of BAC Levels

Most of the intoxicating effects of alcohol occur because of its action on the brain. Alcohol's effects are fairly predictable from the amount in the bloodstream. Therefore, if you know someone's BAC, you can roughly predict what effects alcohol will be having on her or him. Here are some examples:

- Around **20 mg%** light and moderate drinkers begin to feel some subtle effects. This is the approximate BAC reached after one drink.
- Around **40 mg%** most light and moderate drinkers begin to feel relaxed. At this level there is enough impairment of reaction time and fine motor skills that driving is affected. Some countries have already made it illegal to drive at this BAC level. Because there is no truly "safe" amount of alcohol when driving, we concur that ultimately the legal limit should be lowered to 20 mg% (0.02 g%).[15]
- **55 mg%.** At one time, the speed limit nationwide in the United States was 55 miles (90 kilometers) per hour, and this is a reasonable limit for drinking as well. There is good reason to expect that any genuinely *positive* effect of alcohol will already have occurred by the time you reach 55 mg%. Above that level, the effects tend to turn negative. Judgment, perception, learning, memory, coordination, sexual arousal, alertness, and self-control all begin to deteriorate. At the same time, because memory is increasingly affected above this level, you are more likely to remember the effects of lower BAC levels and to forget selectively the less positive later effects that occur at higher BAC levels.

  Any genuinely positive effect of alcohol will already have occurred by the time you reach 55 mg%.

- Around **60 mg%** judgment is impaired. Without necessarily being aware of it, people are less able to make rational decisions

ALCOHOL FACTS: THE MOOD EFFECTS OF ALCOHOL

Many people experience a slight euphoric or relaxing effect at lower blood alcohol levels of 20–40 mg%. Around 60 mg%, however, mood typically falls back to where it was with no alcohol. Furthermore, it appears that the positive mood effects also happen when people *think* they are drinking alcohol, even if they are not. Thus the mood boost may have little or nothing to do with alcohol itself, which is actually a central nervous system depressant.

Above 60 mg%, it's bad news. Mood tends to plunge downward as intoxication increases. There's an odd thing, however. Ask people, after they sober up, how they felt while they were drinking and they often say that they felt happy! It is as though they remember the early effects, but selectively forget what happened to their mood after two or three drinks. And that makes sense, because memory impairment starts to kick in right around the point where mood drops back below the starting point. Bottom line: You get a "happy hour," literally, and it's downhill from there if you drink too fast.

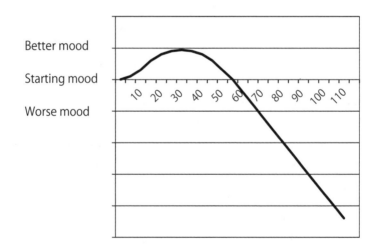

Drinking over time (BAC mg%)

Typical mood effects with increasing BAC.

about their capabilities (to drive, swim, and so forth), and are more likely to take risks they would not take if sober. Learning and memory are also beginning to be impaired at this level. One dangerous aspect of alcohol intoxication is that good judgment is one of the first things to go, and of course it's hard to judge when your judgment has been clouded.

- Around **80 mg%** there is definite impairment of muscle coordination and driving skills. Currently this is the legal intoxication level throughout the United States. Some nations enforce much lower limits.

- Around **100 mg%** there is clear deterioration in memory, reaction time, and the control and coordination of movements.

- Around **120 mg%** vomiting typically occurs, unless this level is reached slowly or the person has developed a tolerance to alcohol. This is the body's first line of defense against overdose.

- At **150 mg%** balance is impaired, and most people have difficulty walking in a straight line. This BAC level means that the equivalent of eight standard drinks (or about 10 ounces [300 ml] of whiskey) is circulating in the bloodstream.

- Around **200 mg%** many people experience a "blackout"—they will have no memory of all or part of what happened during a period of time when their BAC was above this level.

- By **300 mg%** most people lose consciousness—the body's last protection against overdose.

- **450 mg%** is the average fatal dose for adults; breathing and heartbeat stop.

To be sure, there are individual differences in how people respond to alcohol. With enough drinking, for example, people can stretch their tolerance and survive BAC levels of 600 mg% or higher. For youth, on the other hand, a dose of 200 mg% or less may be fatal.

SETTING AN OCCASIONAL LIMIT

Earlier, you established a regular limit for your drinking—the maximum number of drinks for an ordinary drinking day. Now it's time to consider a different kind of limit. Based on the preceding information, what would be the BAC level above which you would choose not to go even on those occasions when you may drink more than your regular limit?

Occasional BAC limit: _____ mg%

We'll come back to this number shortly, but first you need to know how to estimate the BAC level you reach with various amounts of drinking. (Remember that if you are going to be driving, boating, or engaging in other potentially risky activities, we do not recommend any BAC level greater than zero.)

ESTIMATING YOUR OWN BAC LEVEL

Your BAC is determined primarily by four things: how much you drink, how fast you drink it, whether you are female or male, and how much you weigh. There are other factors that do affect BAC levels, such as age, menstrual cycle, and food in the stomach, but you can get reasonably close with just your weight, gender, the number of standard drinks, and the number of hours of drinking.

Appendix C contains a set of computer-generated BAC tables based on sex and body weight. Find the table for your gender (men or women) and closest to your own body weight. Mark that page, because you will be using it more than once. (If you weigh more than 240 pounds [110 kilograms] or less than 100 pounds [45 kilograms], you will have to use those weights. If you're exactly in between [for example, 130 pounds (60 kilograms)], round down [to 120 pounds (55 kilograms)].) You might also want to make a copy of your table and carry it with you. Many of our clients have found their personal BAC table to be one of the most illuminating parts of the program. Many people, for example, have had no idea how the amount they drink converts into blood alcohol levels. These tables give you a specific way to set sensible limits for your drinking and to understand how long it takes for alcohol to be cleared from your body. If you have internet access, you can generate your own personal BAC table at *http://casaa.unm.edu/BACTable/*.

Now you're ready to use your table. Across the top of your table you will see various periods of drinking. This is the length of time (in hours) from starting the first drink to finishing the last. Down the side you'll find the number of standard drinks, ranging from one to 25. Now try these three steps.

Step 1. Watching your BAC rise. On your table, run your finger down the "1 hour" column. As you go from one standard drink to two to three and so on, you can see the BAC level that the computer projects for various amounts of drinking within 1 hour. How much does your BAC level go up with each drink? Try the same for the "2 hours" column.

Step 2. Watching your BAC drop. Next run your finger along the row for five standard drinks. If you had five standard drinks in 1 hour, what would your BAC level be? Now, moving to the right, what if you spread the same five drinks over 2 hours? Over 3 hours? Over 4 hours? How much does your BAC drop with each hour?

This is also how you can estimate how long it would take for your BAC level to get down to zero after having had a certain number of drinks. Suppose, for example, that you had three standard drinks in 1 hour. What would your BAC be, according to your table? Now, assuming you don't drink any more alcohol after that, what would your BAC be after 1 more hour? After 2 hours? How many hours would it take to get rid of all the alcohol from those three drinks? Regardless of how sober you feel, we strongly recommend that you allow your BAC level to drop all the way to zero before driving, boating, swimming, using machinery, or doing other potentially dangerous activities.

Some people are surprised, at this step, to discover that even after they have "slept off" a night of drinking, their BAC is still high the next morning. One mother was shocked to find that she had been driving her children to school with a BAC level well above the legal limit. Had she been pulled over, she could have been arrested for driving under the influence, even without having drunk anything since the night before.

Step 3. Honoring your limit. This is the trickiest step in using your table. Remember the occasional limit that you wrote down just a few pages ago—the BAC level that you choose not to exceed? Now you can use your table to estimate how that limit translates into standard drinks.

Suppose, for example, that you chose a BAC level of 60 as your limit. Take a look at the table for a 180-pound (80-kilogram) male. The total number of drinks this man could have and still stay under a limit of 60 mg% would be three drinks in 1 hour (three drinks would result in a BAC of 46 mg%, whereas four would raise his BAC to 67 mg%). If he spreads his drinks over a period of 2 hours instead of one, he could have four drinks (BAC = 51 mg%) and still stay under his BAC limit of 60. Similarly, he could have only five drinks over 3 hours (56 mg%), and even over a period of 4 hours, six drinks would still put him just over his limit (61 mg%).

Compare the numbers for a 140-pound (65-kilogram) woman. For her to stay at or under a BAC of 60, her limits would be:

Two drinks in 1 hour (48 mg%)
Two drinks in 2 hours (32 mg%)

Three drinks in 3 hours (48 mg%)
Three drinks in 4 hours (32 mg%)

Even a 180-pound (80-kilogram) woman, with the same body weight as the man mentioned previously, would have lower limits than those for the man because of the sex difference in the rate of breaking down alcohol in the stomach:

Three drinks in 1 hour (59 mg%)
Three drinks in 2 hours (43 mg%)
Four drinks in 3 hours (52 mg%)
Four drinks in 4 hours (36 mg%)

Now try it for your own table. For your own occasional BAC limit of mg%, what is the maximum number of standard drinks you could have and still stay within your limit during:

1 hour of drinking?	_____ standard drinks
2 hours of drinking?	_____ standard drinks
3 hours of drinking?	_____ standard drinks
4 hours of drinking?	_____ standard drinks
5 hours of drinking?	_____ standard drinks

We must emphasize that these tables estimate *average* BAC levels for men and women. Of course people do differ from each other, and these tables will not be exactly right for any one individual. Your BAC is influenced by other factors, such as how recently you've eaten, your stage in the menstrual cycle, the mood you are in, your age and the health of your liver, and even your genetic makeup. We certainly can't guarantee what your BAC level will be. Still, these tables are useful in setting goals because they give you a best guess about BAC levels you can expect to reach with different quantities of alcohol. In addition to the amount you drink, they take into account three other important factors: your sex, your weight, and the amount of time you take to finish the drinks.

Notice another important fact: The number of drinks you can consume per hour and still stay within your limit decreases with each hour. Being able to have three drinks in 1 hour does not mean you can have six in 2 hours. Once you're up to your maximum BAC, it takes (for most people) less than one drink per hour to stay there. This is because the liver can break down only a small amount of alcohol each hour, and as you continue to drink the alcohol continues to build up in your bloodstream.

WHAT WOULD YOU GUESS?

Some people are able to "hold their liquor" better than others. They can drink larger amounts of alcohol without feeling or showing the effects of intoxication that most people would have at the same blood alcohol level. What do you think? Are such people who are more able to hold their liquor:

- At less risk of developing alcohol problems and dependence than other people?
- At just as much risk as other people?
- At greater risk of developing alcohol problems and dependence than other people?

The answer is in the "Alcohol Facts" box on page 48.

"Can't I Just Tell from How I Feel?"

In helping people learn how to moderate their drinking, one thing that we tried was to teach them how to know their BAC from their own bodily sensations. We used a breath analyzer to give feedback of actual BAC and had people attend to their own bodily feelings.[16] Some people can learn to do this, but ironically those who need it most seem to be least able to learn it. Heavier drinkers are often unable to learn how to judge their intoxication level from how they are feeling, even with biofeedback and training. In contrast, the estimation methods described in this chapter can work for anyone, regardless of how much they drink.

Sobering Up: True or False?

Is there anything you can do to lower your BAC more quickly or to keep the alcohol you consume from taking effect? Circle "True" or "False" for each of the following statements.

1. Coffee or vitamins or other drugs will decrease the impact of alcohol.

    True   False

2. You will not get as drunk if you avoid mixing different kinds of drinks.

    True   False

3. You won't get as drunk on beer.

    True   False

4. Exercise gets rid of alcohol more quickly.

    True   False

ALCOHOL FACTS: TOLERANCE

People with a high tolerance for alcohol can reach higher BAC levels without feeling or showing the effects that most people would. Some people think that such tolerance—"being able to hold your liquor"— is a special kind of protection or immunity: that those with high tolerance for alcohol are therefore at less risk. Actually the opposite is true. If you can reach high BAC levels without seeming to feel or show it, you're at much greater risk for developing alcohol problems and dependence. It's like lacking a built-in alarm system that most people have. The alcohol is still there in the bloodstream, doing damage to the body and affecting mental functions; there's just nothing to warn you that it's happening. In short, having a high tolerance for alcohol does not protect you from its long-term damage to the body, much of which is related to high BAC levels. The more hours of intoxication (at an elevated BAC level, whether or not you feel it), the greater the damage done.

All of these beliefs are myths:

1. **False.** A stimulant such as coffee does not cancel out the effect of a depressant. Instead, you have a "wide-awake drunk."

2. **False.** What matters is the total amount of alcohol you consume. You get just as drunk on six 12-ounce (350-ml) beers as you would on three beers plus 4 ounces (30 ml) of liquor, assuming you drink them over the same period.

Having a high tolerance for alcohol does not protect you from its long-term damage to the body.

3. **False.** Remember that a 12-ounce can of beer (at 5% alcohol) contains more alcohol than an ounce of 100-proof liquor. A majority of the accidental deaths and injuries, chronic illnesses, and social problems related to alcohol in the United States are consequences of beer drinking.

4. **False.** Exercise does not speed up the rate at which alcohol is eliminated from the body.

Only two things can help to keep you from getting drunk:

1. *Eat before and during drinking.* Having food in the stomach decreases the speed with which alcohol is absorbed into the bloodstream. Drinking on an empty stomach increases the impact of alcohol because it goes directly into the bloodstream and on to the brain. The longer alcohol stays in the stomach, the more it can be broken down before it gets into the blood (particularly in men). Oily foods that coat the stomach (such as olive oil) work best. Huge doses of fructose (fruit sugar) do speed up alcohol metabolism, but you're unlikely to be able to eat enough fruit to make a difference. Certainly a fruit juice mixer won't save you.

2. *Drink moderately.* This is, of course, the surest preventive measure against intoxication.

From now on, use your table when you want to estimate your BAC. If your weight changes substantially, switch to the table nearest to your new weight or generate a new one from *http://casaa.unm.edu/BACTable/*.

Remember Your Limits

One of the first things people usually try in managing their drinking is to set specific limits for themselves. Actually, that is a good first step. This chapter was designed to help you set sensible limits, informed by knowledge about drinking and how alcohol affects people. Now put them all in one place, using the Personal Goals Card on page 50 (or make a card of your own). You first set a regular limit (page 40), the number of standard drinks that you chose as your upper limit for most days when you drink. What was it? Record it on your Personal Goals Card.

Then you also selected a BAC level that you choose not to exceed on

PERSONAL GOALS CARD

My regular limit: _____ standard drinks per day

My occasional BAC limit: _____ mg%

          _____ standard drinks in 1 hour

or _____ standard drinks in 2 hours

or _____ standard drinks in 3 hours

or _____ standard drinks in 4 hours

or _____ standard drinks in 5 hours

From *Controlling Your Drinking* (2nd ed.). Copyright 2013 by The Guilford Press.

occasional days when you may go over your regular limit (page 44). Write your occasional BAC limit on the Personal Goals Card.

Finally, using your table from Appendix C, you translated this into a maximum number of drinks you would have in various lengths of time and still remain within your occasional limit (page 46). Record these on your Personal Goals Card.

> A 34-year-old construction worker, Adam, came to our clinic for help in managing his drinking. He had been divorced for 6 months, and over that period of time his use of alcohol had increased steadily. Several times he had been involved in fights while drinking on weekends. A few weeks before coming to the clinic, he had been arrested for driving while intoxicated. This was the first time he had ever been arrested, and the experience upset him.
>
> Adam was drinking an average of 50 drinks per week, including about 36 glasses of beer and 14 mixed drinks. He tended to have five or six drinks a day, mostly after work with the guys. On weekends he drank more heavily, both at home and when he went out to bars. Following the step-by-step procedure for setting limits, Adam first decided that he should set his regular limit at three drinks per day. He was surprised to learn (in the "How Many Adults Drink That Much or More?" table on page 39) that only 3% of American men drink as much as he had been drinking. He also considered the recommended drinking limits for avoiding harmful effects of drinking in the long run. He thought about setting his regular limit at two drinks per day, but that seemed a pretty big change from his current

pattern. That's why he picked three drinks as his limit, thinking that down the line he might want to reduce it further to two.

For his occasional limit, Adam decided that he wanted to keep his BAC within the "speed limit" of 55 mg%, maybe allowing himself "five miles over." So he set his occasional limit at 60 mg%. Then he used his BAC table to translate this into a number of standard drinks. He located his weight table (180 pounds [80 kilograms], Appendix C, page 264) and he looked down the columns for 1, 2, 3, 4, and 5 hours until he came to 60 (or the closest level under it). Using this method, he found that he could stay under his limit if he had:

Three drinks in 1 hour
Four drinks in 2 hours
Five drinks in 3 hours
Five drinks in 4 hours
Six drinks in 5 hours

To simplify this, he decided on two drinks in the first hour and one per hour after that. He was curious, too, about what his BAC would be when he had his regular limit of three drinks. He calculated (by using his table) that if he drank his three drinks within 1 hour, his BAC would be 46 mg%. If he had the same three drinks over a period of 2 hours, his BAC would be only 30 mg%. If he spread them out over 3 hours, and had one drink per hour, his BAC would reach only 14 mg%. Finally, if he distributed three standard drinks over 4 hours (or had them in 3 hours and then waited 1 more hour), his BAC would be zero. (This is true because Adam's body could keep up with this rate of drinking, processing virtually all of the alcohol as he drank.) Together, these limits seemed reasonable to Adam. It would be challenging, to be sure: He had to cut his drinking in half at least, but he thought he could live with no more than three drinks a day on most days and could have at least one day a week without drinking at all. (Saturdays, he thought, because that was the day he got to spend with his kids.) The plan still allowed him to go over the regular limit by a drink or two now and then, while staying within the safety net of his occasional limit.

About 3 weeks down the line, Adam found himself resenting his limits. He had been reasonably successful in sticking to his regular limit on most days and had exceeded his occasional limit only once, but he began to feel trapped. Why did he have to stop at three drinks? Who said he couldn't have more? That kind of mental claustrophobia is common when observing new limits. It can feel as though you've been deprived of some freedom. Adam had been talking to himself about how unfair it was to have these limits (see Chapter 19). But then he answered his own questions. Why did he have to stop at three? In fact, he didn't have to. He had chosen to, and there were good reasons for his choice. Who said that he couldn't have more? There was no one else policing him; he had set his own limit. If someone else had set the limit for him, it would have been easier to rebel, but again he realized that the limits were his decision, his own choice, and he reminded himself of the good reasons for his choice. He also realized, though he hated to admit it, that he was feeling a good bit better in the morning, particularly on Mondays.

For Adam, the regular limit was useful in cutting down his total amount of drinking. His occasional limit was also important, though, because he had tended in the past to drink to very high BAC levels, especially on weekends.

Becky was a college senior who had heard about our self-control program through a psychology class she had been taking. It appealed to her because Becky was someone who liked to be in control and in charge. She was a popular person and a reasonably good student, although her drinking had interfered with both her studies and her friendships at times during college. She was particularly worried because at a recent party she had blacked out while drinking and had no memory of the latter part of the evening, including how she got home. She also worried because her father had had problems with drinking when he was younger and had quit drinking about 10 years ago.

In an average week, Becky consumed about 25 standard drinks, mostly beers. She tended to have most of them in one or two evenings, mainly on weekends. On other days she drank little or nothing. This had been her pattern since high school, although the amount she drank had been increasing in recent months as graduation approached.

Becky followed the steps for deciding about limits for her drinking. She wasn't so concerned about a daily (regular) limit, because on most days she didn't drink at all. She knew from experience, however, that when she did drink on weekends, her judgment gradually eroded. That was what she particularly wanted to avoid. She noticed on the BAC information that this impairment usually occurs around 60 mg%. To stay under this, she chose 50 mg% as her upper limit for BAC on any occasion.

Then she went to her own BAC chart (120 pounds [55 kilograms],

Appendix C, page 253) to find out what her drinking would need to be like to stay within a 50 mg% limit. She was surprised:

> *One drink in 1 hour*
> *Two drinks in 2 hours*
> *Two drinks in 3 hours*
> *Three drinks in 4 hours*

Not even one drink per hour! She considered loosening up a little, setting a higher BAC level as her occasional limit so she could have a few more drinks. She was used to having eight beers or so in the course of a weekend evening, which, she discovered, explained why she couldn't remember some of the time. She also learned that she had often been driving with a BAC well over the legal limit. "Why not give 50 mg% a try?" she thought. She could always change her mind later.

For Becky, her regular limit was less of an issue. Except on weekends, she usually had one or at most two beers or glasses of wine. It would be no problem, she thought, to make it a rule that except on special occasions, she would have just one drink on days when she drank. It was those special occasions that she had to be careful about!

Before moving on, take one more look at the goals you've set for yourself. Do they seem reasonable? Is that what you want to shoot for, at least for now? If so, give it a try! You're free, of course, to revise your goals upward or downward later.

Once you have clear goals set for yourself, the next challenge is how to stick with them. *Everything else in the chapters that follow is designed to help you reach your goal of self-control within these limits.* It's up to you to decide how best to reach your goal, choosing from the menu of methods that we suggest or trying out your own ideas. There is a pleasant side to this responsibility, too. Any change that occurs in your drinking is clearly your own accomplishment. Success in using self-control methods is *your* success. That's why it's called *self*-control.

Chris was a 46-year-old suburban mother. Her husband, an attorney, was often gone for long hours, and her two children had recently moved away. She had been drinking almost every day, mostly glasses of wine at home alone or with neighborhood friends, for several years. Her consumption had gradually increased to about 40 drinks per week, including drinking with housework, meals, and during the evening.

Chris decided that her regular goal would be to drink no more than one glass of wine. The occasional limit she set for herself allowed a maximum of three drinks within 4 hours. She carefully determined the one-drink (4-ounce [125-ml]) line on her wine glasses, so as not to kid herself and overpour.

Within 2 weeks Chris had become totally discouraged. She had failed to stay within her regular limit on 13 out of 14 days. She felt like giving up her self-control program altogether. We advised her to try setting a more liberal limit for herself, at least temporarily.

Chris did adjust her limits. She set a regular limit of two drinks for the average day. She changed her occasional limit only slightly, to four drinks in 4 hours. This seemed to help. She went over her regular limit only twice during the next 3 weeks and exceeded her occasional limit on only one day. Encouraged by this progress, she wanted to tighten her limits again. We suggested that she continue with the more liberal limits for another week or two, which she did. Eventually, she went back to a regular limit of one glass of wine per day. She bought more expensive wine, sipping and savoring her daily glass. For occasional days when she decided to go over her regular limit, she kept to a simple safety-net limit of three drinks per day.

By adjusting her limits, Chris avoided becoming so discouraged that she would give up completely. Through her more reasonable limits (which she viewed as a step along the way), she gradually accomplished her original goal. Every step toward moderation is a step in the right direction!

5

•

Keeping Track

To learn most any skill or accomplish any intentional change, you need at least two things: a clear goal and accurate feedback about how you're doing. Chapter 4 focused on the goal. Now it's time to give yourself reliable feedback. It's very hard to practice archery in the dark: You may shoot a lot of arrows, but you're not likely to get much better at hitting the target unless you can see where your shots land. Learning requires good feedback. That's what this chapter is about.

This step is fairly simple. You need to start keeping track of your drinking—keeping good records of your alcohol use, much as you would use a checkbook (or, these days, software) to keep track of your use of money. As with a checkbook, keeping good records is far better than occasionally thinking about what you've done and trying to guess how you are doing. When you keep good track of your drinking, you know for sure. Psychologists refer to keeping track of what you do as "self-monitoring."

There are three good reasons to start self-monitoring now.

1. First and foremost, you need accurate feedback. When you count your drinks, you know for sure whether you are moving in the right direction. It's right there in black and white, and there is no fooling yourself about it. Either you are moving toward your goal or you are not.

2. Self-monitoring in itself seems to help people reduce their drinking. When we asked people who succeeded with our program what they had found to be most helpful, the one thing they most often mentioned was keeping these records. They said things like

"It helped me be more aware of my drinking, to pay attention."

"The cards caused me to think about it each time before I took a drink."

"Keeping these records, I couldn't kid myself. It was right there in front of me."

3. The self-monitoring method described here also leads to self-discovery, helping you learn more about your own drinking. When you get to Part III, the records you have kept will be very useful in helping you analyze the situations in which you tend to drink too much.

Remember that this is *self*-monitoring—something that you do yourself, for yourself.

So what is involved in self-monitoring? It requires carrying with you a small card and something to write with, much as people keep a running record card when they play golf. If you carry with you and use an electronic device that lets you keep records, so much the better. The system that we recommend for keeping track of your drinking looks like the form below.

You can make a simple version of this on standard 3" × 5" lined index cards just by writing a few words across the top and drawing vertical lines to divide the columns. Lined index cards are available in office supply, stationery, and discount stores, as well as many supermarkets and drugstores.

Daily Record Card

Date	Time	Type of drink	Amount	Situation

From *Controlling Your Drinking* (2nd ed.). Copyright 2013 by The Guilford Press.

Find a simple way to make yourself a supply (by photocopying onto card stock, printing from a computer, and so forth), because you may be using quite a few of them in your self-control program.

Then get used to carrying your record cards around with you all the time. Put them in a convenient place such as your pocket, purse, checkbook, or wallet. You'll also need a pen or pencil to write with (unless you're using an electronic device). Once you've done this, you are ready to start self-monitoring.

How to Use Self-Monitoring Cards

The rule for effective self-monitoring is fairly simple: *Every* time that you have *any* alcohol beverage *anywhere*, write it on your card *before you drink it*. As the card illustrated here indicates, there are five things to write down, at least in abbreviated form, each time you have a drink: the date and time, the kind and amount of the drink, and something about the situation in which you are drinking. Now for the practicalities.

Know What You're Drinking

To keep good records of your alcohol use, you have to know what you are drinking. In particular, you need to know how much alcohol there is in the drink in your hand. That requires that you know two things: how many ounces of beverage you have and what percentage of alcohol it contains.

OUNCES

When you are drinking a beverage from a commercial can or bottle, the number of ounces is usually indicated on the label. In the United States a can or bottle of beer is usually 12 ounces, but they do vary in size from small "stubbies" to large cans and bottles of 40 ounces or more. A fifth of wine is one-fifth of a gallon, or just over 25 ounces (about six standard drinks at 4 ounces each). Liquor tends to come in pints (16 ounces), fifths, or quarts (32 ounces). If you happen upon metric units, you can convert liquid measures into ounces:

1 liter (1,000 ml) = 33.8 fluid ounces
1 fluid ounce = approximately 30 ml, which means that
1 standard drink (½ ounce) = 15 ml of ethyl alcohol

It becomes a little trickier when beverages are poured into a glass. If there are certain glasses that you tend to drink from at home, fill them up as you usually do and then pour the contents into a measuring cup (minus any ice if you use it). When pouring distilled spirits, use a measuring cup. A shot glass is OK if you know how much it contains when filled to the line or rim. Bar glasses vary quite a bit in size, but your server or bartender will know how much alcohol it contains. If you feel a little self-conscious, there are low-key ways to ask this. For example, you could say: "I'm driving—could you please tell me how much alcohol is in the margarita?" Most servers and bartenders are concerned about their customers' safety and will be glad to give you accurate information. Avoid "topping up" your glass, because that makes it harder to keep track of how much you are drinking. Just put your hand over the top and say "No thanks" until you've finished the drink you have. (If you're afraid of appearing rude, some ideas for refusing drinks courteously and comfortably are explained in Chapter 8.)

PERCENTAGE

The other thing you need to know is how much alcohol the beverage contains. In the United States, manufacturers of wine and liquor are required to list on the label the amount of alcohol the beverage contains. For wine, this is usually listed as a percentage of alcohol content, which for table wines is usually somewhere between 9% and 14%. If you have to guess with a table wine, use the average of 12%. However, some wines, called fortified wines, are stronger. These include port, sherry, brandy, and cognac. Again the alcohol content varies, averaging around 20%. Check the label.

With a few exceptions, distilled spirits (liquor) tend to contain between 40 and 50% alcohol. The term "proof" in the United States is a number that is just double the percentage of alcohol, so that 86-proof whiskey contains 43% alcohol, and 100 proof is half alcohol. Sipping liqueurs vary widely, but again the alcohol content must be specified on the label.

That leaves beer. So far, U.S. manufacturers and distributors have not been required to specify how strong a beer is in terms of alcohol content. Most standard brands in the United States contain about 5% alcohol, so as an average that is a reasonable guess. Some (but not all) light beers contain less alcohol than that (about 4.2%), and certain brands can contain 10% alcohol or more, overlapping with wines. You can find the strength of your favorite brands, along with calories and carbs, on websites like *www.alcoholcontents.com/beer/beer.htm*.

A real problem emerges if you have a drink of unknown strength, such as when someone mixes it for you in another room or you drink a punch of unknown content. In general, it's best to avoid this situation. Ask to mix your own drink if that's possible or watch it being done. Find out how much of what beverages are in the punch bowl or avoid mystery punches altogether.

WRITING IT DOWN

As much as possible, it's best to have about one standard drink at a time. Some examples of this would be a 10-ounce glass of beer, a 4-ounce glass of wine, or about an ounce of distilled spirits. If you're writing down amounts like these:

Type of drink	*Amount*
Beer	Quart
Beer	6-pack
Wine	Liter
Vodka	Pint
Whiskey sours	5

you're drinking too much at a time, and chances are you're writing it down afterward. Break it up into one-drink units, and remember to write it down just *before* you start each drink.

When and Where

Notice that in addition to type of drink and amount, the daily record card has columns for other information to be recorded. This information includes:

> *Date:* the date on which you are having the drink
> *Time:* the time of day when you take the first sip of the drink
> *Situation:* for keeping track of special information that may be impor-
> tant in your drinking (This is discussed in more detail in Chapter
> 11. For now, just ignore this last column.)

With a little practice, you'll be able to write all this information on your card or in an electronic device within a few seconds.

It's important to get into the habit of writing this information down *just before* you take the first sip of your drink. If you do it this way, the record keeping helps you be more aware of your drinking. If you wait until later to write down the information, you'll be losing much of the potential benefit of this self-control method. If you end up not finishing a drink, you can always change the entry.

It's important to get into the habit of recording the information about your drink just before you take the first sip.

It can be a bit of a challenge to keep track while you're drinking, but this is an important first step in getting a handle on your use of alcohol. If you have trouble getting started with faithful record keeping, here are some things that people have done to remind or motivate themselves:

- Make it a rule never to take a drink before recording it, and think of the first sip as your reward for writing it down.
- Figure out a good reminder for yourself—something you'll see just before you drink and that you can use to remind yourself to keep notes. Some possibilities are a small stone in your pocket or a card in your billfold that you will see when you reach for money; a note in the display on your cell phone (use a code word if you don't want to announce what you're doing to anyone who sees your phone); a ribbon on your bottle; a note on your refrigerator; a special glass or coaster that you use when drinking.
- Each time you write down a drink before starting it, say something encouraging to yourself, such as "Good for you," or "Way to go," or "I'm really sticking with my program."
- Involve other people in your record keeping. Someone you trust can help you remember to write down your drinks and can encourage you to do so. Don't ask this person to *police* you—it's your responsibility to keep the records—but it can be helpful if someone else knows what you're doing and encourages you.

Like most habits, once you get into the pattern of writing down every drink before you start it, it becomes easier and more natural.

"What If Someone Asks Me What I'm Doing?"

Some people are very comfortable writing down their drinks around other people, but others are concerned about how those around them might react

Personal Reflection

With diabetes, I have to keep pretty close track of what I eat to manage my blood glucose level. After years of measuring sugar levels in my blood by prick-ing my fingers with a test kit, I have a pretty good grasp of how to keep my sugar levels lower. But sometimes I get careless about keeping track. I figure I know what I'm doing, and stop checking my sugar levels. Then there's a part of me that thinks I can get away with pushing the limits, and if that goes on for a while, I might even think, "Maybe I don't really have diabetes." But it's just as lawful as gravity, and I'm only kidding myself if I don't keep track.

—WRM

to their record keeping. Our experience has been that most people don't even notice the cards, or they think nothing of it. It's even less noticeable if you keep your records in a small notebook, a checkbook, or an electronic device.

What can you say, though, if somebody does happen to notice and asks what you're doing? There are no answers that work for everybody, but here are a few of the replies people have used:

"I'm trying to cut down, and I'm keeping track of my drinks."
"I'm on a diet, and I'm keeping track of carbs."
"I'm keeping track of expenses."
"It's something I'm doing for myself."
"It's something I'm doing for a class."
"I'm taking notes for the FBI."

Be creative and see what you can think of to say! Usually a short answer is enough and a long explanation is unnecessary.

Another alternative, if you're in a situation in which you don't want to have to answer questions, is to be more subtle. Here are some creative ways that people have managed to keep their records when they didn't want to answer questions:

- Excuse yourself to go to the rest room or make a call and jot down your entry in private.
- Leave the table and go to the bar when you make your notes.
- Make a notation on your bill, bar tab, or charge slip.

Many people find self-monitoring easy and interesting. Most had never really paid that much attention to counting and spacing their drinks or estimating their own BAC level. Remember that it takes only a few seconds to write it down. The important thing is to figure out a way to write each and every drink down *at the time*, just before you take the first sip. Otherwise you're compromising on an important self-management method.

Some Personal Experiences in Self-Monitoring

None of the methods we use has produced more comments and stories from our clients than this process of self-monitoring. A few of these experiences may be helpful as you get started with your own record keeping.

CALLING HOME

Some years ago, one woman was very self-conscious about keeping records. She always drank with friends and didn't want to have to answer any questions about what she was doing and why. At first, she went to espionage-like lengths to conceal her self-monitoring. She lived alone and had voice mail on her phone, which recorded the date and time of all incoming calls. When she was out with friends, she used her cell phone to call home at the time she was starting a drink. (Now she would probably be sending herself text messages.) Because she always had the same drink when she was out, she didn't have to remember what kind of alcohol it was. When she got

---

KEY STEPS FOR EFFECTIVE SELF-MONITORING

1. Keep a card and pen or pencil with you at all times, unless you're keeping electronic records.
2. Write down *each and every* drink before taking the first sip.
3. Record the type of drink, amount, date, and time of first sip.
4. Record one drink at a time.
5. If you do, on occasion, fail to record a drink, do it later. Better late than never!
6. Use a card until it's full and then begin a new card, or you can start a new card each day if you wish. What matters is having complete and accurate records of your drinking.

home, she would retrieve the call times from her voice mail and transfer them to her record card with the exact time of each drink, also noting where she had been and with whom. After a while, though, she tired of this method, and she was also having to make up stories about the calls she was placing. She then switched over to jotting down the times in a little notebook that she carried in her purse and found that this raised no suspicion. If she felt self-conscious, sometimes she would go to the ladies' room to make her notes in the privacy of a bathroom stall. She also observed that the inconvenience of recording each drink seemed in itself to have slowed down her drinking.

EXTERNAL MEMORY

One fellow was particularly conscientious about recording every drink just before the first sip, with accountant-like accuracy. The record keeping became so linked to each drink that soon he didn't even have to prompt himself to keep records. He didn't care who asked or who knew what he was doing. He just told them the truth—that he was keeping track of his drinks. One woman he was dating commented, "I do that with what I eat!" and they joked about their record cards all through dinner. He was still drinking quite a bit during his early weeks of self-monitoring, and he observed that "It's sure good I'm keeping these records, because otherwise I'd have no idea how much I drank." One morning he woke up fuzzy-headed and found he couldn't remember part of the night before. He recalled the first couple of hours, but after that it was a blank. He pulled out his self-monitoring cards, and there they were: drink-by-drink records of the evening, right through his period of blackout! He could even estimate the BAC level at which he stopped remembering, which sure enough was just over 200 mg%.

STRUGGLING

Another person had trouble keeping her records. She intended to keep them, but something always seemed to get in the way. She didn't have a pen, she left her cards at home, or she just got caught up in conversation and forgot about it. At other times she felt embarrassed or resentful about writing down her drinks. Usually she did try to remember to write them down on a sheet of paper after she got home or the next day, but she found she had trouble reconstructing exactly what she drank when. After 5 or 6 weeks of this, she was getting discouraged and was ready to give it all up.

That's when she had a little flash of realization. "This is so easy, and yet I've been dodging doing it. I'm trying to convince myself that it's just too hard to do, but that's not it. I'm dodging taking an honest look at my drinking." She went back to review why she was doing this program in the first place (Chapter 2), and something just clicked. After that, she said, it was suddenly easy for her to keep records!

Your Weekly Summary of Progress

As we've pointed out, the daily record cards can be valuable in several ways. One of these is that they help you keep track of your progress in managing your drinking. Even small steps toward moderation show up! To really appreciate your progress over a period of weeks, though, you need a way to summarize and interpret your cards. For this purpose we provide a Summary of Progress form (see below). This form is straightforward. You simply fill in one column every week, making an entry in each of the six lines. We suggest that you begin keeping cards on a Monday so that your recording weeks end on Sunday. Make entries on your Summary of Progress form every Sunday evening. You may copy the form provided here or make your own.

Using the Summary of Progress can do at least two things for you. It will mean, first of all, that you'll be sitting down at least once a week

Summary of Progress Form

Week ending (date):					
Total number of drinks this week:					
Number of days I stayed within my regular limit:					
Highest number of drinks in any one day this week:					
Number of hours spent drinking on highest day:					
Estimated highest BAC level this week (use BAC table):					

to evaluate your progress. This self-evaluation will be based not on vague recollections (as when you wait until the end of the week to recall your drinking) but on accurate information about your actual drinking pattern. Using the summary form can also provide encouragement. There is no better reward for using self-control methods than to see yourself making progress toward your goal. If your self-management program is succeeding, you will see your gradual progress on the cards and on your Summary of Progress.

David was a 38-year-old sportscaster for a local TV station. He entered the self-control program because of his concern that his drinking could cost him his job. More and more often he had been going to work still feeling the effects of his previous night's drinking. David began the self-monitoring portion of his program by purchasing a pack of 3" × 5" lined index cards. He made up 20 cards with the five columns shown in this chapter. David always carried a pen and notebook in his pocket, so he simply folded one card and put it with his notebook. He folded an extra card and placed it in his wallet, in case he filled up the first card while he was away from home.

On Monday morning David began keeping records of his drinking. He worked that day and had two beers during lunch. He was feeling a little nervous about keeping the records, so he wrote down the first beer by going into the men's room. The second beer was part of a round that he bought, so he recorded it when he went over to the bar to order.

On Monday night he went to his favorite weeknight spot. There he met a group of friends and joined them. They quickly poured him a glass of beer from the pitcher on the table. Determined to stick to his recording, David managed to write it down without being noticed. When his glass was half empty, a friend picked up the pitcher and started to refill glasses. David put his hand over the glass and said "That's OK. I'll get some more in a minute." To his surprise, no one asked about his refusal. In fact, no one even seemed to notice in the midst of the conversation.

Three glasses later a friend happened to notice the card and asked, "Hey, Dave, what are you doing?" Everyone turned to see what he was doing.

Dave was ready. "Well, I'm keeping track of what I drink this week," he said. "I'm on a kind of diet. Besides I'm curious about how much I can put away in a week."

"Hey, you're gonna need a book!" said one of his friends. They all laughed, and the conversation went on to other topics. After that no one paid any attention to his cards.

David found that when he started keeping daily record cards, it seemed as if he drank less. It was a little inconvenient to keep the cards, but he was interested to find that something so simple could make him more conscious of his drinking.

One week David slipped up. He stopped keeping track of his drinking one night and began writing it down only at the end of the day. It seemed just as good to him. When Sunday came around, however, he noticed as he filled in his Summary of Progress that he had had more drinks than usual and had gone over both his limits. That was with the drinks that he had written down, and he was sure that he had forgotten several more. He decided to go back to writing drinks down just before the first sip.

Altogether David used daily record cards for about 6 months, until he had his drinking down to a level that satisfied him and was confident that he could keep it there. For him, the record cards themselves seemed to be what kept his drinking level down.

We recommend that you begin keeping daily record cards as soon as possible. You don't necessarily have to make any changes in your drinking right away. You could keep records for a week or two to get a rough idea of your average drinking rate and to provide a starting point from which to reduce your drinking.

Record keeping itself seems to move many people toward moderation.

Don't be surprised, though, if the record keeping itself seems to move you toward moderation. Many people find that just keeping records makes them more keenly aware of their drinking. On average, people using this program reduced their drinking by about a third when they began self-monitoring, which can be a very good motivational head start.

6

•

Taking Charge

Now that you've set limits for yourself (Chapter 4) and you've learned a method for keeping track of your progress (Chapter 5), you're ready to begin trying some methods for changing your drinking.

As indicated in Chapter 5, it's a good idea just to keep records for a week or two. Once you get used to keeping track of your drinking, you can start to use the self-control methods described in the chapters that follow. In essence, we're offering you a menu of things to try.

Whenever you begin a self-management program, it is tempting to try everything at once. We urge you to take it easy and try one new technique at a time. Some will probably work better for you than others, and by trying them individually you can discover the ones that work best. The one-at-a-time approach also allows you to concentrate on each method and to practice it until it feels natural to you. Take a good look at the menu and then decide what to try next. For example, if other people who push drinks on you are a big problem, maybe Chapter 8 is a good place to start. In looking through the "slowing down" ideas in Chapter 7, you may find one or two that particularly appeal to you. Give them a try. People who succeeded with this program didn't use every last suggestion. Rather, they told us that they found a few things that worked best for them and stuck with those.

When you're ready, begin with the methods presented in Chapters 7, 8, and 9. These chapters explain things you can do when you are drinking that often can have a relatively quick effect in reducing your drinking. Try out these methods and then continue to use the ones that work for you while you add new skills from Parts III and IV.

The methods explained in Part III of this book add ways to plan control over your drinking. Experiment with the methods described in these chapters, continuing to use the "when you drink" skills from Part II.

Chances are that some of the chapters in Part III will be more relevant to you than others.

Finally, go on to Part IV. These chapters explore some common motivations for overdrinking and suggest alternatives to the use of alcohol in each case. Once again, some chapters will apply to your situation better than others will. Give special attention and effort to those chapters that deal with factors that seem to be important in your own drinking. If, for example, you tend to drink when you feel "down," you might give priority to Chapter 21. If you drink to fall asleep, Chapter 23 may be helpful.

Changing habitual behavior is a gradual process. Mark Twain observed: "Habit is habit, and not to be flung out the window by any man, but coaxed down-stairs a step at a time."[17] Take your time and add new methods as you feel comfortable with previous ones. As the weeks pass, reread sections of this book and try out new techniques. Once a week, perhaps every Sunday after you fill in your Summary of Progress form, briefly review what worked well for you and what didn't. If you found a certain technique somewhat helpful but think maybe you could get more out of it, reread the section that introduced it. If your review has pointed out areas that are problematic for you—for instance, you find that you're more likely than you realized to drink too much in certain situations—turn to the sections in Part IV that describe strategies aimed at them. In this way, you can learn to use self-management methods and can add them to your permanent storehouse of personal abilities.

People who succeeded usually picked a few methods that worked well and practiced them faithfully.

In the end, you're likely to find a few methods that seem to work particularly well for you. When we followed up with people who succeeded in using this book, they usually had identified a few methods that worked well for them and practiced them faithfully. The key is to find, from the menu of options that we offer, the ones that work for you.

Rachel was a reasonably steady drinker. Mostly she drank light beer at home or with friends. When she began keeping record cards, she found that she was averaging six or seven a day, which she knew was less than she had been drinking before she started self-monitoring. The record keeping made her more conscious of how much she was drinking. She was also surprised to learn that the particular German "light" beer that she preferred contained almost as much alcohol (4.8%) as regular beer. She'd been telling herself that she wasn't really drinking that much because it was light beer.

Through the process of goal setting, she chose limits for herself that amounted to no more than one light beer per hour, with a maximum of three per day. That meant slowing down considerably from her past drinking habits. After reviewing the ideas in Chapter 7, she came up with two that seemed likely to work well. Mostly she relied on clock watching—writing down the time when she started each beer and not starting another one until an hour had passed. That meant making a beer last longer. At first she tried taking smaller sips and putting the beer down in between, but she soon found she didn't like this method because the beer would get warm, and she liked it cold. When at home, she tried pouring about half of the beer into a chilled glass and keeping the rest of the bottle in the refrigerator to keep it cold, but that seemed like too much of a hassle. What worked for her was to sip more slowly, making the beer last longer, and then having something else to drink in between. She settled on club soda because it is carbonated and has no calories. She also began to try "near beers" with almost no alcohol and found that she enjoyed them. With those changes, she made clock watching work for her.

In reflecting on triggers for overdrinking (Part III), Rachel knew immediately what characterized those occasions on which she really overdid it. It was when she was with a man who drank a lot and who encouraged her to keep up with him. In this situation she began using a few of the lines from Chapter 8 to refuse drinks that would take her over her limit. And of all the material in Part IV, Rachel found the ideas on "talking to yourself" (Chapter 19) to be most natural, as she already did a lot of internal talking to herself. She could easily imagine using her stubbornness and telling herself such things as "Stick to your limit, Rachel. This guy is just trying to get you drunk."

Together, these tools worked well for her. Within a few weeks she was sticking to her limit and, on most days, having just two light beers. She also experimented with having only the club soda on some days, and she particularly enjoyed doing this when she was out with friends, just to see their disbelief. Then just when they thought she had become a teetotaler, she'd have a beer. Rachel liked to be a little mysterious and keep them guessing.

7

·

Slowing Down

One of the simplest ways of staying within the limits that you've set for yourself is to *slow down* your alcohol consumption. Most people who drink too much do so in part because they drink too fast. Because it takes a little while for alcohol to exert its effects, they may be feeling the second drink while they're having their fourth or fifth. Consequently, they become convinced that it takes four or five drinks to get the effect they like. Then, unfortunately, drinks number three, four, and five take effect. One person told us, "When I feel like I want another martini, I just wait 20 minutes and I feel like I've had one." Think of alcohol as an over-the-counter drug. If you choose to use it, you need to learn which dose produces its beneficial effects and when you are overdosing.

If you feel like you want another martini, wait 20 minutes and you'll feel like you've already had one.

Another good reason to slow down is to adjust your tolerance to alcohol. As we explained in Chapter 4, tolerance (being able to "hold your liquor") is usually not a good thing. You need ever larger doses of alcohol to experience the same effect, but your body still has to process it all. As one person observed, "If I could get a six-beer buzz on just three drinks, that would be great. But if I have to drink six beers to get the same buzz that I used to get from three, then I'm at a point of diminishing returns."

Alcohol tolerance adjusts to how much you drink. Even having one drink decreases your response to the next drink. It's that fast. When you drink more, your tolerance increases. As you cut back on drinking, your tolerance decreases.

This chapter suggests some ways of slowing down your drinking, the second step toward moderating your drinking.

Types of Drinks

People who have problems related to drinking often tend to order and consume *stronger* drinks. By "stronger" we mean that the alcohol content is high. Here are some relatively strong drinks:

Malt liquor and ale
Martinis
Liquor, straight or on the rocks
Doubles
Fortified wines: sherry, port, muscatel, vermouth

There's more alcohol in malt liquor than in regular beer; more alcohol in all-liquor cocktails, such as martinis and Manhattans, than in those with an alcohol-free mixer, such as highballs or screwdrivers; more alcohol in straight liquor than in mixed drinks; more alcohol in doubles than in a single shot; and more alcohol in fortified wines than in regular wine. Consequently, if you have these stronger drinks, you will become intoxicated (that is, your BAC will rise) much more quickly than if you had been drinking their lighter alcohol counterparts.

One simple but effective way to slow down your alcohol intake, then, is to switch to drinks that are not so strong, that have less pure alcohol in them. Some *less concentrated beverages* are:

- Mixed drinks (instead of straight liquor).
- Low-alcohol beers—but don't be fooled: "light" beer doesn't necessarily mean it contains less alcohol.
- Table wines (normally 12% alcohol) instead of fortified wines. Again, check the label. Wine manufacturers are required to tell you the alcohol content.

By selecting less concentrated beverages, you'll be taking in less ethyl alcohol per sip. If you're unfamiliar with these beverages, educate yourself! Experiment with different kinds of drinks. Break out of the habit of "the usual." Browse through a recipe book for mixed drinks, read up on wines, try ordering and buying new and less concentrated beverages.

Another tip about types of drinks may be helpful. Some drinks are very tasty, and it's easy to drink them fast. These include blender drinks and sweet fruity beverages such as sangria, punch, mojitos, and tropical cocktails.

There are also plenty of people, however, who overdrink on less concentrated beverages like beer and table wine. Most likely there are beverages that you tend to drink more quickly than others. Probably your favorites fall into this category. Become aware of the drinks you tend to gulp and try some alternatives. Try switching to drinks that have unusual or even less pleasant tastes for you. (Make sure, though, that any unpleasantness is not the sting of concentrated alcohol!)

Eve, a 26-year-old counselor, dearly loved Riesling. She always ordered it when she went out to a restaurant or lounge, and she kept a supply at home. In examining her drinking, she realized that when she was offered other kinds of drinks, she usually tended to sip them more slowly. This was particularly true of dry red wines and drinks made with soda water. Eve tried drinking dry Chianti and cabernets and found that she did indeed take longer to finish them. After a few weeks, she became familiar with a range of different wines and practiced sipping them slowly, savoring the tastes. When ordering mixed drinks, she selected ones made with soda water. Her slower sipping made the drinks last longer and substantially decreased her total alcohol consumption. Eve also found that she grew to like the taste of dry wines and of mixed drinks. (People usually learn to like whatever they drink, perhaps because the pleasant effects of alcohol or the pleasant circumstances of drinking become associated with the taste of the drink. Then, of course, you have to be careful not to start drinking these faster!)

You may protest, "But I really *like* the taste of my favorite beverages!" Yes, of course you do! It may just be helpful to switch beverages in managing your drinking. This is especially likely if your favorite drinks have a high alcohol concentration and you switch to beverages with lower alcohol content. Most Americans who overdrink, though, do so with beer, so it's not just a matter of drinking beverages with less alcohol in them. You, like Eve, will probably find that you grow to like the beverages to which you switch. Know and enjoy a range of beverages, and don't stick to one "favorite." The key here is to use the beverages that make it easiest for you to drink them slowly and in moderation.

Making It Last

There are some things you can do with any drink, including your favorite, to make it last longer. Basically, these things have to do with sipping.

Try counting the number of sips that it takes for you to finish a drink. Don't attempt to change it at first. Just sip in your normal manner, but keep count. Then try to increase the number of sips you can get out of a drink. This means, of course, you will have to take smaller sips. We recommend you get at least 12 sips (and preferably more) out of each drink. Try it! If you have drinks with ice, try adding more ice about halfway through.

Taking smaller sips won't do you a bit of good if you compensate by sipping faster. It's also important to space your sips. Allow at least a full minute (and preferably more) between sips. If there is a second hand on your watch or on a clock nearby, you can practice spacing out your sips and get the feel of it. Try leaving longer intervals between sips. Don't feel obliged to sip every 60 seconds! What is it like to allow 90 seconds to pass without sipping? Two minutes? When you're first practicing this, you might record the number of sips per drink on your daily record card and examine how long it takes you to finish each type of drink. Be particularly careful with the first sips of a drink, because that's when people tend to drink the fastest.

One simple trick that helps is to put the drink down and take your hand away from it in between sips. It breaks the habit of holding and sipping. Beware of drinking absentmindedly, which can happen, for example, when watching television. The discipline of slowing down your pace of drinking involves mindful awareness, at least at first. You're changing a well-established habit.

> At 55, Phillip, a high school teacher, was drinking primarily at home. He drank mostly scotch, of which he polished off 2 to 3 quarts (2 to 3 liters) per week. He came to our program under pressure from his family and his principal.
>
> The process of self-monitoring startled Phillip somewhat. He purchased his scotch by the case, which had protected him from immediately confronting how much he was drinking on a daily basis. Keeping records in itself helped him decrease his intake a bit, but it was clear that his well-established drinking habits needed to change.
>
> When Phillip began paying attention to his pace of drinking, he noticed that the word "sip" didn't exactly describe what he did. He tended more to gulp his drinks. It took him three or at most four gulps to finish a drink, and he was pouring another one within a few minutes. He decided to try taking smaller sips and to sip more slowly. He watched the second hand on his watch and sipped only once a minute. In between sips, he put his glass down. This felt strange at first, but using this method, he found that his

drinks began to last much longer. With the glass out of his hand, he sometimes got involved in something else and did not sip for several minutes. Still, he was getting only six or seven sips per drink.

Phillip decided to switch from drinking his whiskey neat to having it on the rocks. At first the ice made it seem watery, but he still enjoyed the taste. Ice cubes made from pure spring water seemed to enhance the aroma. Moreover, he was able eventually to get 10 to 15 sips out of one scotch, and his drinks were lasting 20 minutes or longer, especially when he was involved in something else that used his hands. He collected puzzles that challenged him, such as old Rubik's cubes of various sizes, so he kept some of these on the coffee table to fiddle with while he was drinking and found that it helped him take a longer time between sips. He also enjoyed the puzzles and began adding to his collection.

Spacing Your Drinks

The basic idea behind drink spacing is to decide that you will have only one drink within a certain amount of time. This means setting another limit for yourself: a time limit.

As an example, refer back to the occasional BAC limit that you set for yourself in Chapter 4. To stay within your blood alcohol concentration limit, what's the maximum number of drinks that you would consume within *4 hours?*

Write it here: _____ drinks in 4 hours

Now divide this number into 240 (the number of minutes in 4 hours):

240 minutes / _____ drinks = _____ minutes per drink

The answer gives you the number of minutes you would need to allow *per drink* to maintain the occasional BAC limit you have set for yourself. Allow *at least* this much time per drink, especially after your first drink.

Now refer back to your *regular* limit. How many drinks is that for an average day? And how many minutes or hours do you spend drinking on a typical day when you drink?

Write it here in minutes: _____ minutes spent drinking in an average day

Now divide this number of minutes by your regular limit (drinks per average day):

_____ minutes ÷ _____ drinks per day = _____ minutes per drink.

This second answer represents the *average* recommended length of time, in minutes, that you would allow per drink.

To summarize the calculations you have just finished:

What is the *shortest* length of time in minutes that you should allow per drink according to these limits? (This is usually the first answer, unless the second answer happens to be smaller.)

Write it here: at least _____ minutes per drink

And what is the *average* amount of time in minutes that you should allow per drink according to these limits? (This is the longer of the two, usually the second answer.)

Write it here: _____ minutes per drink, on the average

Note that moderate social drinkers usually take at least 20 to 30 minutes to finish a drink and take longer per drink after finishing the first one or two. Your goal for average drinking time should probably not be less than 30 minutes per drink (that is, not more than two drinks per hour). See the box on page 76 for examples of the result of faster and slower drinking.

Moderate social drinkers usually take at least 20 to 30 minutes to finish a drink and take longer per drink after finishing the first one or two.

Do these time limits seem reasonable? If not, what do you think would be reasonable time limits per drink? If you drank at this rate for 4 hours, what would your BAC be? (Use your BAC table to figure it out.)

The spacing of drinks, or "clock watching," is one of the most commonly used methods in our program, perhaps because of its simplicity.

If you can gradually space your drinks farther apart, you are moving toward moderation. Also, if you can stretch out your first drinks, you have a good head start. For people who overdrink, a common pattern is to have a few drinks in rapid succession. Slowing down the first drink or two sets the pattern for moderation.

ALCOHOL FACTS: SLOWER IS BETTER

It's a simple fact that the faster you drink, the higher your blood alcohol level will go. Overdrinking (like overeating) is often the result of taking in too much too fast. It is particularly common to drink too quickly during the first hour or so. Consider the example in the graph below, which shows blood alcohol for a 160-pound man who starts drinking at around 5:00 P.M. When drinking "faster" he has three drinks in the first hour, two during the second hour, and then levels off at one drink per hour. By 7:00 his blood alcohol concentration (BAC) is already over 80 mg%, and it continues to rise to 108 mg%. By slowing his consumption to one drink per hour, he keeps his blood alcohol level under 40 mg%.

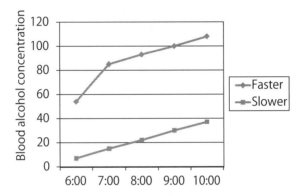

Faster and slower drinking for a 160-pound man.

The second graph below shows the result of the same drinking patterns for a 140-pound woman. For reasons discussed in Chapter 4, her blood alcohol level goes much higher than the man's (in the preceding graph) with the same amount of alcohol. Limiting her consumption to one standard drink per hour makes a big difference in her intoxication level, though even so her BAC goes over 80 mg% after 5 hours.

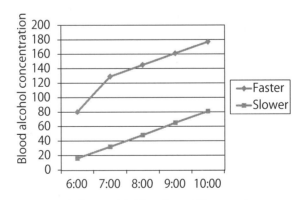

Faster and slower drinking for a 140-pound woman.

Probably your limits indicate that you need to start spending more time per drink. How can you do this? Here are some suggestions:

1. Make your drinks last longer by sipping more slowly and by taking smaller sips.
2. Allow time to pass between finishing one drink and starting the next.
3. Have an alcohol-free beverage between drinks. (This helps if you feel pressured to order something or if you want to have something to hold and sip.)
4. If you like your drink chilled, keep it fresh by adding ice or by keeping it cool (instead of gulping it so that it won't get warm). Wine can be kept cool in an ice bucket, a beer in an insulated can holder.
5. Do something else in between drinks. Have something healthy to eat (and watch out for salty or spicy snacks that make you thirsty). Chew gum. Dance. Talk to someone. Do something that you enjoy.

Gloria was a very busy woman. At 40, she was a successful realtor and the mother of two teenagers. She had found that alcohol seemed to make her hectic days somewhat more relaxed and her more routine tasks less annoying. A series of life stresses had accelerated her drinking, however, and she was occasionally missing appointments. This "irresponsibility" and her increasing impatience with her daughters alarmed her and brought her to our self-control program.

Gloria was a rapid drinker. She spent an average of 10 minutes on a drink and typically poured another as soon as she finished one. It was clear that spacing her drinks more widely would be an important step in self-control.

She began by calculating time limits for herself. Her occasional limit for 4 hours was six drinks. Since 4 hours equals 240 minutes she found that her shortest time per drink should be 40 minutes.

Next she used her regular limit of two drinks per day. She estimated that she spent about 2 hours, or 120 minutes (2 × 60), drinking in the average day. She divided 120 by 2 and found that on the average she should take 60 minutes per drink.

Thus for Gloria to maintain her self-control limits, she should spend 40 to 60 minutes per drink. This seemed an awfully long time to her, but she decided to try it.

She increased her average number of sips per drink from four to about

10. *This helped a lot, making her drinks last for about 20 to 25 minutes. The remaining time she spent either without a drink, sucking on the left-over ice in her glass, or with a soft drink. She found that when she had a soda between drinks, she had no trouble at all in allowing 40 minutes per drink. These simple strategies reduced Gloria's consumption of alcohol, both when she was alone and when she was with others. As her drinking decreased, she found other ways to relax when things became hectic. (The relaxation method she used is described in Chapter 18.)*

8

Refusing Drinks

All your self-management planning can go right out the window if you don't resist drinks offered by others. To keep your agreement with yourself about limits, you, not other people, need to be in charge of what you drink. This means being prepared to refuse offers and even pressure to drink. This pressure can be subtle. Even if no one directly pressures you to have another drink, you may find yourself "keeping up" with those around you. It takes some conscious effort to avoid being swept along in the tide.

Often you can avoid unwanted drinks without even saying a word. If someone picks up a bottle or pitcher and moves toward your half-empty glass, just putting your hand over the top or nonverbally waving the person away is usually enough. If you're leaving a table for a few minutes, you can take your nearly empty glass with you. Leave the table just before a new round is ordered. Order a soft drink. If you find an unwanted drink in front of you, you can just leave it there. In some cultures, in fact, this is how your host knows when you've had enough.

> **WHAT WOULD YOU GUESS?**
>
> Imagine a round table with people drinking together. Which do you think would have a bigger effect on how much people at the table drink: adding one person who drinks very slowly or adding one person who drinks very quickly? _____
>
> The answer appears on page 81.

How you verbally refuse drinks will vary, of course, depending on who is doing the offering. You would probably say different things to a stranger than you would to an employer. It is up to you to craft some lines to handle situations like this. Here are some that other people have used:

"No, thank you."
"Not right now, thanks. Maybe a little later."
"No, thanks. I'm fine."
"No, thanks. I want to wait a few minutes."
"No, thanks. I just finished one."
"No, thanks. I'm on a diet."

Friends will usually honor statements like this, and that will be the end of it. Sometimes, though, you have to respond to additional pressure. Someone might say, "Oh, come on!" or "Hey, what's the matter?" or "Right—now what can I get you?," or even "Can't you handle it?" You should be prepared to cope with this kind of added pressure and not let it undermine your self-control. Here are some second-round lines that others have used successfully in situations such as this:

"No, really, I'm fine."
"Hey, look—not right now, OK?"
"My doctor told me that I need to take it easy, and I'm cutting down."
"I'm really trying to cut down, so how about helping me out?"
"Hey, don't take it personally! I just don't want another one right now."

You can add a light touch or turn the attention back to the drink pusher with a question:

"Am I falling behind here in a race?"
"You're really in a hurry for me to get drunk!"
"Why is it so important to you that I drink more?"
"What is it about 'no' that you don't understand?"

It can be useful to practice your refusing skills before you need them. Ask a friend to pressure you and try out different ways of responding. Make sure that when you do drink, it's because you have chosen to, and not because it's something that someone else asks or wants you to do.

Practice your refusing skills before you need them.

> ### ALCOHOL FACTS: WHO SETS THE PACE?
>
> It's no surprise, perhaps, that the people you drink with can strongly influence how much you drink. What may be more surprising is that this influence seems to work mostly in one direction. In naturalistic research in a bar, psychologist John Reid found that regular patrons' drinking increased substantially when a friendly, fast-drinking male stranger sat down next to them. In contrast, a slow-drinking stranger had virtually no effect on customers' pace of drinking. Several other studies have confirmed this finding: add one fast-paced drinker to a table and everyone else's drinking tends to speed up. Add a slow-paced drinker to a table and it has no significant effect on others' drinking.

Still another way to avoid extra drinks is not to put yourself in pressure situations. Don't go out with a group you know is going to be drinking hard and fast. Leave the party after the first hour. People who make successful changes in their lives often start by avoiding temptation and the harder situations. Those who quit smoking, for example, often avoid other smokers for a while. Then with time, as they become more comfortable in their new identity, they find it easier to be in more challenging situations without violating their limits.

This can be difficult if your friends or family are mostly heavy drinkers. It often happens that over the years people tend to gravitate toward companions whose drinking is similar to their own. You may find, then, that as you moderate your own drinking, you're out of step with the people around you.

We have, of course, often encountered this obstacle in working with people who want to cut down or quit drinking. For some, their entire social network has consisted of heavy drinkers. They therefore seemed to face a choice between continuing to drink too much or being lonely and isolated. The situation is not really so black and white, however, and there are options. Here are some of the things that can work:

- Explain what you are doing to some of your close friends and ask for their help. Get together with them in nondrinking situations.
- Strengthen relationships with people who are not heavy drinkers. We find that often there were friendships and other relationships that people had let go of as their drinking increased. Are there

people you *used to* enjoy being with who weren't heavy drinkers? Look them up.

• Try out new groups and activities that don't require drinking (see Chapter 20). There are plenty of enjoyable people and pursuits that don't involve alcohol. Try them out. There is more about this strategy in Part IV of this book.

Finally, there is one more person whose offers of drinks you can learn to refuse: yourself! You may be aware of a little voice inside you that says, "Oh, go ahead—have another one. It won't hurt." Though it may sound odd, you can also talk back to that voice inside, often with the very same lines that you might use in refusing a drink from someone else. There is more about talking to yourself in the next chapter, as well as in Chapter 19.

WHAT'S A PARTY?

Italy had just won the World Cup, and there was mayhem in the streets of Rome. Pedestrians simply took over the streets: dancing, shouting, singing, and waving Italian flags. Surprised to see no one drinking, an American tourist asked, "Why aren't you partying?" making the hand-sign for drinking. A festive Italian replied, "Who needs to drink when we're having so much fun already?"

9

•

Affirming Your Progress

At this point you've set specific goals for yourself (Chapter 4), and you've developed a way to measure your progress by keeping track of your drinking (Chapter 5). You've learned some ways to slow down your rate of alcohol consumption (Chapter 7) and considered ways of resisting offers and pressure to drink (Chapter 8). In short, you've chosen a destination and are considering how best to get there. It's a journey that can take a while. The familiar saying that "a journey of a thousand miles begins with a single step" is true enough, and it continues with thousands of small steps after the first one.

Anyone who is progressing on a long quest can use some encouragement along the way. Give *yourself* some encouragement! One good reason for keeping the Summary of Progress form (Chapter 5) is to recognize and celebrate your progress on the journey, even small steps. Congratulate yourself when you're making progress toward your goal! Talk to yourself! (It really isn't crazy.) If you stayed within your limits on 5 days out of 7, affirm those 5 days instead of just criticizing yourself for the other 2. Recognize where you've done a good job in managing your drinking and affirm even minor changes in the right direction. Most progress is gradual. Reminding yourself that you're making progress (when you are) can help you continue your gradual successes.

*Hannah, a 29-year-old employee of the telephone company, enjoyed going to parties and going out with friends for "a few drinks." It was to enjoy a **few** drinks that she came to the self-control program.*

Hannah knew that one of the hardest things for her was refusing drinks. Men were always buying her drinks, usually before she had even finished the previous one. She practiced how to refuse drinks by having a close friend pressure her, and soon she had developed a few lines that felt comfortable and natural for her ("That's sweet, but not right now, thanks"). In social settings she found herself more and more able to accept drinks only when she wanted them.

Every time Hannah successfully refused a drink that she didn't want, she said to herself something like "Way to go, Hannah! You refused that drink well. Not only that, but you did it in a way that made him feel good about having offered!" This self-affirmation made her feel good about her ability to manage her own drinking. When, on occasion, a refusal offended somebody, she would still talk to herself affirmatively. "That's OK. You did the right thing. You really didn't want that drink, and you refused it nicely. It's his problem if he can't handle it."

Another possibility is to congratulate yourself with some tangible reward. Think of it as a celebration of your success!

Not just any old reward will do. Usually the most effective rewards are those that (1) are tailor-made for you, (2) can be enjoyed as soon as possible after your success, and (3) are "extras." Let us explain what we mean.

• **Tailor-made rewards.** What is rewarding for you may not be rewarding for another person. That's one reason it's best for you to choose your own rewards. Watch out for specific details that can make an intended reward backfire. An afternoon in the country may be very satisfying— unless you happen to suffer from hay fever. Food is an unwise reward if you're trying to lose weight. And of course drinking is not a good reward for reducing drinking.

Here are some guidelines for choosing rewards that are tailor-made for you:

1. They should be pleasant enough that you would really work to earn them.
2. They should be brief enough that you can afford the time.
3. They should be inexpensive enough that you can easily afford the cost.
4. They should be varied enough so that you don't get tired of them.

• **Available rewards.** A second quality of good rewards is that they are easily available. A good reward is something you can enjoy almost any-time. Food treats are a common example. You can keep a snack around, ready to be eaten anytime you earn it. Buying a magazine at a supermarket is a bit less available as a reward, but you could do it the same day you earn it. A trip to a national park is not very available and may be too distant a reward to encourage your daily successes. A distant reward like this may be a good final celebration when you've completed a long-term project, but it is important to also reward small steps along the way to your goal.

One way to make distant rewards work for you on a daily basis is to give yourself points. To reward yourself with a massage, for example, you could set the "price" of a massage at, say, 50 points. As you achieve minor steps toward your goals, you earn points toward your massage. The same principle can apply to items such as clothing, a new piece of sports equipment, or a CD or DVD recording. Similarly, as you decrease your drinking, you can save up the money you *would have* spent on alcohol until you have enough to buy something that you really would like. This has sometimes been referred to as "turning alcohol into furniture."

- **Extra rewards.** Good rewards are tailor-made and available. A third thing that makes a reward attractive is an "extra" quality. By this we mean that it is above and beyond the rewards you normally experience. Part of the benefit of using rewards to reinforce your progress is that you bring more positive experiences into your life. If you reward yourself with things that you would have had anyhow, it's not exactly a reward. Suppose you enjoy surfing the Internet and often spend an hour doing so. If you decide to use that hour as your reward and then fail to earn it, you're depriving yourself of even your usual pleasure. It's much better for rewards to be extras—activities or things that you wouldn't ordinarily have and that bring you extra pleasure.

"Not Me! I Don't Need Rewards!"

Some people don't think they should reward themselves. "I don't need payoffs," they say. "I shouldn't have to be paid to do what I ought to do anyway. That's childish!"

The fact is that we all need and use rewards. We do what we've learned to do, and we all respond to incentives. Through the careful use of positive reinforcement, you can change your own behavior. Why not give yourself this extra encouragement to make the changes you want? Make it easier for yourself to change and enjoy some well-deserved celebration along the way!

We all need and use rewards—think of them as a celebration of your success.

Some Ideas for Rewards

Having trouble thinking of what to use as incentives for yourself? Here are some suggestions divided into two types: material and mental.

Material rewards usually require an expenditure of money or time or both. Some material rewards that require money or time are:

1. *Objects:* Magazines, music, books, cosmetics, clothing (the truly tailor-made reward), games, gadgets, furniture.
2. *Food:* A nice meal, special treats, sweets, bakery items, ice cream, fancy special dishes, tropical fruits such as mangos, papayas, or fresh pineapples.
3. *Stepping out:* Movie, restaurant, dance, play, museum, park, exhibit, fair, shopping, a tour.
4. *Miscellaneous:* Money for a special cause, a gift for a friend, money for a special savings account.
5. *Social time:* Time with people to talk, play games, go somewhere, converse on the phone, kiss, make love, walk, run.
6. *Sit-back-and-appreciate time:* Time for concentrating on something that is interesting to you; listening, reading a book, watching TV or people, reading letters, Internet surfing.
7. *Do-my-own-thing time:* Time for those things that you "never have time to do," such as painting, drawing, sculpting, potting, putting, puttering, writing, building something, playing an instrument, working on your car or sound system, putting together a model or a puzzle.
8. *Do-nothing time:* Time when you don't have to do anything. Waste it. Rest. Daydream.

Mental rewards are things that you imagine or say to yourself. They can be compliments about something you've done or about some characteristic of yourself that you value. In other words, as discussed earlier, mental rewards involve saying something positive to yourself about yourself. Some mental rewards for something you did might be:

"I really did a good job today."
"What I did for her really helped her."
"I handled that situation well."
"That was pretty hard, and I finished it on time."

"It took some doing to refuse that drink, but I did it."
"Getting up on time today was really an accomplishment."
"I practiced good self-control this week."

Some mental rewards concerning your personal characteristics might be:

"I'm dependable."
"My family really cares for me."
"I'm smart."
"I work hard and play hard."
"I'm sensitive."
"I'm honest."
"I'm attractive."
"I'm competent. I know what I'm doing."

Still another kind of mental reward involves imagining something pleasant. After accomplishing a goal, you reward yourself by picturing a very positive scene. You might imagine yourself relaxing on a summer beach, walking in a cool forest, or enjoying some other setting. A good way to do this is to see yourself reaping the natural benefits of your self-control. For example, when you're successfully managing your drinking, picture yourself:

Waking up without a hangover and feeling good.
Having lost some weight.
Having more friends.
Buying something you've wanted with the money you've saved.
Being healthy and spry at the age of 85.
Having a happier love life or family life.
Getting a clean bill of health after a checkup.
Doing well at your work; getting a promotion or better job.

If you're saving up points or money for a special celebration, such as a massage or a trip, you can also imagine it already happening.

Both kinds of rewards, material and mental, are important. Both have their advantages. Material rewards are good because they are tangible and can be a source of extra positive experiences in your daily life. A material reward makes a kind of celebration. Mental rewards are useful because they can be used anytime, anywhere. They can be totally tailor-made because they come directly from you and because you can give them to yourself as soon as you accomplish a goal.

Personal Rewards

Take a few minutes now to think of some good rewards for yourself. Start with material rewards. What things could you afford (in terms of money or time) that would be pleasant? What would you work for? Remember that better rewards are those that are easily available (a special sandwich, not a new home). What are some material rewards tailor-made for you? Think of at least five and write them here:

_____

_____

_____

_____

_____

Now think of some possible mental rewards for yourself. What things might you say to yourself? Write here at least five statements that say something positive about you:

"_____"

"_____"

"_____"

"_____"

"_____"

"_____"

Write at least five positive things that you could say when you've done something well:

" _____ "

" _____ "

" _____ "

" _____ "

" _____ "

" _____ "

Making an Agreement with Yourself

Now that you've considered how to choose rewards for yourself, here's how to go about setting up a simple "congratulations" agreement:

1. *Decide what would be a reasonable amount of progress for you.* What would you regard as a successful next step? Don't be too hard on yourself. Small increases in self-management count. It helps to set up a series of small steps for yourself. For instance, if you wanted to lose weight, you might reward yourself for each pound lost rather than waiting until you reach your final goal.

2. *Choose a reward* that you will give yourself when you have taken your next step. Try both material and mental rewards.

3. When you have a goal (Step 1) and a reward (Step 2), *make a commitment* that if you do make the progress that you set for yourself, you'll congratulate yourself with the reward(s).

4. Use your daily record cards to *determine whether or not you achieve your goal.* If you don't, decide whether you may be trying to take too big a step at one time.

5. *Reward yourself when you succeed.* If you miss your goal, don't reward yourself. Rewards will not help you change if you get them no matter what you do.

Manuel was worried because his drinking had begun to interfere with his work as a medical technician. He had made some significant errors that had been called to the attention of his supervisor. In addition, he had some problems with his stomach, and overdrinking usually resulted in annoying pains. The physical discomfort had already reduced his drinking somewhat, but he wanted to cut back further.

Manuel had been consuming about 30 drinks per week. He decided on a regular limit of 12 drinks per week (no more than two a day, and 1 day a week without alcohol) and made this his goal. He made a contract with himself that involved a series of small steps, extended over 6 weeks. The steps were:

First week: decrease drinking to 27 total drinks.
Second week: decrease drinking to 24 total drinks.
Third week: decrease drinking to 21 total drinks.
Fourth week: decrease drinking to 18 total drinks.
Fifth week: decrease drinking to 15 total drinks.
Sixth week: decrease drinking to 12 total drinks.

This program would get him to his regular limit within 6 weeks. That seemed reasonable. Next he thought about what he could use as a reward. It should be something he really liked, something extra that he could deny himself if he did fail to reach a goal. He decided that using more data with his cell phone would be a good self-reward. Manuel loved music and liked to stream it and then share the best of it on Facebook. Going over the limit on his data package was expensive, but it still seemed like doing that periodically would cost him less than committing to a much more generous data plan every month. He decided that if he made his goal for a week, he deserved to use the data he wanted on that Sunday.

This was Manuel's agreement with himself: "If in the first week I don't have more than 27 drinks, I can use my phone all I want on Sunday. If I go over 27 drinks, I won't use my phone for anything but calls and texts that day."

Manuel used his daily record cards each week to determine whether or not he had made his goal. He did make his goals for the first 3 weeks and connected with a lot of friends on Facebook through the songs he shared, which he really enjoyed. Then in the 4th week he had one night of overdrinking, and his total for that week was over his goal of 18. Because he had been enjoying the Sunday data usage, he thought about using his phone for whatever he wanted anyway, but he decided to stick with his agreement. He decided to keep the same goal for the next week, and he did stay below 18. That Sunday night he streamed some music videos that he loved, which made him feel great—and so did his continuing progress.

Partners in Progress

You may wish to involve someone else in your self-management contracts. If you do, it should be someone you trust, who will not use it as an opportunity to criticize or nag you. It should be a person who is genuinely interested in your well-being and in helping you reduce your drinking. For one woman we saw, the most supportive person was clearly her mother, with whom she had a close and warm relationship. "She's always there for me and always tries to build me up instead of criticizing me." This mom had the ability to be supportive without being overinvested. For others whose parents are more prone to advice giving and criticism, mom or dad might not be the best choice. One man chose as his partner a friend who used to be part of his hard-drinking group but who had pulled back to spend the time with his family. A brother, sister, coworker, or pastor might be the right person. It also doesn't have to be someone you see in person. Some have preferred to use a supportive friend who lives far away, staying in touch by telephone, e-mail, or social media.

There are at least two ways in which a partner can help you:

1. A partner can be interested in and encourage your progress, discussing it with you at regular intervals (once a day, once a week, and so forth). You might share this book with your partner and together come up with strategies. Mostly, though, it's helpful just to have someone to talk to as you work on changing your drinking. He or she doesn't have to have brilliant ideas or try to fix problems for you. In fact, tell your partner you just want him or her to listen as you share your experiences. Stephen, for example, confided in his brother Paul about his drinking and his efforts to moderate it. He hadn't told his brother about it before, but Paul wasn't surprised. In fact, he was relieved because he had been silently worried about Stephen's drinking, and he felt good that his younger brother had confided in him. Paul wanted to do whatever he could to help and sometimes went a little overboard with advice, but mostly he listened. They established a pattern of texting each other every day and talking by phone a couple of times a week. Paul would text "How many?" around the same time each night, and Stephen would text back the number of drinks he'd had that day. Just knowing he'd have to tell Paul helped him, even though they had agreed that Paul would neither praise nor criticize Stephen. He'd just text "Got it" to confirm receipt. When they talked on the phone, Paul would check on how his brother was doing and encourage him when he got down on himself about a slip-up.

2. A partner could share in the rewards you give yourself. Your part-ner could actually give you the reward, or you could enjoy it together (or both).

Suzanne was an adventurer. She had in her younger years enjoyed camp-ing with friends, rock climbing, white-water rafting, and especially four-wheeling in the desert. As her drinking had increased over the past few years, however, she had stopped doing these things and had lost touch with her more active friends. When she thought about who might be her part-ner in progress, she immediately thought about her friend Lydia, whom she hadn't seen for some time. Her phone number was still the same, and Lydia was surprised and glad to hear from her. Yes, she still had that old Jeep. Suzanne explained her situation, and Lydia was sympathetic and ready to help. In fact, going out four-wheeling together again would be fun.

There are at least two ways in which you should not use a partner:

1. Don't put another person in the role of police officer. If you make someone else responsible for keeping you honest, you may easily fall into some destructive patterns of relating. You're responsible for managing yourself. This is a particular danger when your partner in progress is a loved one.

Sam chose his wife as his partner in progress, as he had already confided in her and she certainly knew about his overdrinking. Soon, however, he fell into an adolescent-like pattern of trying to outsmart her, to "get away with" drinking without her knowing about it. She knew him well, though, and after three incidents in which he had been less than honest with her about his drinking, they both decided that it wasn't good for her to take this role. As his new partner in progress he enlisted a buddy from work, an "older and wiser" guy who wasn't part of the drinking crowd.

2. Don't have your partner penalize you if you fail to reach a goal. Being deprived or penalized by some-one else does not help you feel good about that person. In addition, you could be tempted to deceive in order to avoid the consequence. Set up your agreement so that you're responsible for change and the other per-son's role is one of encouragement and positive rein-forcement.

Don't ask a partner to police you or to penalize you.

Here are some guidelines if you wish to involve a partner in your contract:

1. Choose someone whom you trust and who cares about you. This should be someone who isn't too emotionally tied up with your drinking and also who is not a heavy drinker.

2. Tell him or her about your goals and plans and show your partner this book.

3. Explain that you're not asking this person to be responsible for your progress, only to be interested in it and you.

4. Explain clearly how the person can help. Tell your partner specifically what you want him or her to do and not to do to support you. Can your partner help with or share in the rewards you give yourself? How will you keep your partner aware of your progress and struggles? When will you discuss your progress? How will your partner encourage you?

Judy and John had been married for 8 years when he was arrested for driving under the influence. He had been drinking at home alone when the beer ran out, and he decided to drive to the supermarket. On the way back, just a few blocks from home, he ran a red light and narrowly missed causing a crash. His car wound up on the sidewalk against a light pole, and within minutes the police had arrived and he was in handcuffs.

John was surprised that his BAC registered 120, particularly because he didn't feel at all intoxicated. In beginning this program, he was eager to read his BAC chart, which did indeed predict that given the six beers he had consumed, his BAC could even be a bit higher—about 125. Obviously he had been far more intoxicated than he realized.

Being handcuffed, fingerprinted, and jailed was humiliating, and John wanted to make sure it would not happen again. He first used his BAC chart to find out what he needed to do to make sure there was no alcohol in his body before getting behind the wheel. Then he set his two limits: a regular limit of three beers on most days and an occasional BAC limit of 60 mg%, which translated into three beers in 2 hours or four beers over 3 hours. Even on "special" occasions, he decided, three would be his limit. It was a simple rule to follow.

There was no question in John's mind who his "partner in progress" should be. Judy had already been concerned about his drinking even before his arrest. They were definitely still in love, and there was no one he trusted more than Judy. He told her about his program and goals and asked for her support, which pleased and touched her.

The first thing they thought of, jokingly, was no sex on days when he went over his limit, but that was a penalty for both of them rather than positive reinforcement for John. Judy was happy and relieved that John wanted to moderate his drinking and was willing to look for some special celebrations for those weeks when he stayed within his goal. Together they came up with a short list:

Cook a favorite meal together
Go out to a movie
Share a hot bath together (no alcohol)

They agreed that during weeks when John made his goal, he could pick the menu that weekend. She wondered at first if he would be completely honest with her, as often he drank when she was out. Her worry faded, though, as they looked over his record cards together, and she also saw clear changes in his drinking, mood, and attentiveness to her. John didn't meet his goal every week, but they shared a lot of meals, movies, baths, and fun along the way on the many weeks when he did.

10

•

Moving Along

Congratulations! You've finished Part II, on things you can do *while* you drink. Next we turn to some things that you can do *before* you drink to maintain moderation.

Before going on to Part III, however, take stock of your progress thus far. Here are some questions to help you check your understanding and use of the material in Part II. If you cannot answer "Yes" to any one of them, go back and review that chapter:

- Have you set a clear regular limit for yourself? Do you know what it is? (Chapter 4)
- Do you know what BAC means? (Chapter 4)
- Have you set an occasional BAC limit for yourself? What is it? (Chapter 4)
- Do you understand the difference between your regular and your occasional limits? (Chapter 4)
- Do you know how to make and use daily record cards? (Chapter 5)
- Have you decided how to respond to people who ask what you're doing when you're using the cards? (Chapter 5)
- Do you have a clear plan for how to make drinks last longer? (Chapter 7)
- Do you know how far apart to space your drinks to stay within your limits? (Chapter 7)
- Are you prepared to deal with pressure to drink? (Chapter 8)
- Have you worked out a system for rewarding your successes, including a set of gradual weekly steps toward your goal? (Chapter 9)

Are you ready to go on? Here are some questions asked frequently at this point in the program.

How long should I go on using the daily record cards?

Obviously you're not going to use them for the rest of your life. Their purpose is to help you get your drinking down to a moderate and safe level and to increase your awareness of your drinking pattern. We definitely recommend that you use the cards for at least 10 weeks or until you have your drinking at a level that satisfies you and have kept it there for 3 or 4 weeks. In other words, keep records until you have met your goals and your new drinking pattern is stable. If at a later time you find that your drinking has increased again, it may help to resume the use of self-monitoring cards.

How long should I continue using the other self-control methods from Part II?

Here we can say "for the rest of your life." This program is not like a diet that you go on temporarily to lose weight. Rather, the methods described here represent a moderate *style* of drinking that you would continue to practice as long as you want to keep drinking in moderation. They involve a change in your everyday habits. Actually, the same is true of diets. Temporary and crash diets are usually unsuccessful in taking weight off and keeping it off. Stable weight loss involves establishing everyday patterns of choosing, preparing, and eating foods.

> *Keep records until you have met your goals and your new drinking pattern is stable.*

Should I be using all of the methods from Part II?

Not necessarily. The point is to use *enough* of them to reduce and stabilize your drinking at your goal level. As indicated previously, we strongly recommend that you keep careful records of your drinking during this period of change. Think of this as a period of trial-and-error experimentation. Try out methods for slowing down drinking, spacing drinks, refusing drinks, and such and see how they work for you. Particularly stick with the ones that do help you moderate your drinking.

How soon should I see a change?

In our studies, most people who succeeded in moderating their drinking made substantial reductions within about 6 weeks. On average, they cut their drinking at least in half during this time. People working with this book continued to reduce their drinking over a period of 6 months, after which it didn't (on average) either decrease or increase much. So you should be seeing good progress within 6 to 8 weeks. Our experience with this program is that if it hasn't produced a good reduction in your drinking within 10 to 12 weeks, it's not likely to do so later. At that point, it would be time to try something else. There are many options, as discussed in Part V.

Should I change my drinking by a certain amount before going on to Part III?

Not necessarily. You ought to have completed at least a couple of weeks of self-monitoring and be trying out specific methods for reducing your use of alcohol. The methods from Part II are necessary but may not be sufficient to moderate your drinking. Once you're applying the methods from Part II, go on to Parts III and IV for additional ideas that may help you manage your drinking.

Is there anything I should watch out for at this point?

It can happen that as you decrease your use of alcohol, you increase your use of another drug. That is, you substitute one drug for another. By "drug" we mean to include tobacco, prescription medicines (such as tranquilizers and sedatives), and over-the-counter medicines (such as sleeping aids and aspirin), as well as consciousness-altering illicit drugs. If you use any of these substances, be mindful of the extent to which you are using them as you work on reducing your drinking. We find that most people do not, in fact, increase other drug use when they cut down on drinking, but be alert to this possibility.

As you cut down your drinking, you may also encounter things that you've been using alcohol to cope with or avoid. Part IV of this book particularly focuses on these issues. If you feel physically ill as you cut down, see your doctor. We also provide some guidelines in Part IV as to when you should consider seeking professional help.

What if it's not working for me?

It may be a little early to tell at this point. We urge you not to give up too quickly. It often happens that a person making progress in self-control will have some setbacks. If you do happen to overdrink and exceed your goals, get right back on your program the next day. There is no point in beating up on yourself about it. Most people who have successfully moderated their drinking have still had occasional days of excess.

But what if you do try, honestly and patiently, and still find that your drinking has not changed? What if you continue to have too many over-drinking days and alcohol-related problems? What then? That is why we have added Part V to this book. If you continue to struggle with modera-tion after 10 to 12 weeks, it's time to read the concluding chapters of this book. They will help you consider whether abstinence may be a more fea-sible goal for you.

Part III

●

Before You Drink

In Part II we discussed things that you can do *while drinking* to increase your self-control. This section focuses on things that happen *before you drink*—what precedes or triggers your drinking.

A first step is to discover what your own triggers are, the topic of Chapter 11. Chapters 12 to 16 then go into the individual kinds of triggers in more depth and offer suggestions for what you can do about them.

As with Part II, try out the methods we describe. *Don't just read about them*. Experiment with them to find out which ones work for you. Some chapters may be particularly important, whereas others address topics that are simply not an issue for you. Find out what really makes a difference in your drinking and then focus on those methods.

11

•

Discovering Your Triggers

It's 5:30 in the afternoon, and Kirk has just finished a particularly bad Monday. The loss of several more clients has driven his monthly sales to a new low. Driving home, he sees a bar he hasn't visited before and decides to stop for a "quick one."

This is a bar in which some regular customers drink rather heavily. As the evening crowd shuffles in, the bartender turns down the lights, and someone buys a first round.

Kirk is feeling very low. He is tired, hungry, thirsty, and discouraged. He sits down on a stool next to one of the regulars, who is rapidly downing shots of whiskey.

Kirk is in trouble. There are several aspects of this situation that make it very likely he is going to drink too much. He's weary and moody. It's 5:30 and his stomach is empty. The people around him are drinking heavily. The atmosphere is dark and private. He's thirsty. People are buying rounds. All of these are frequent triggers for overdrinking.

Perhaps you've noticed that in certain situations you tend to drink more, whereas in other situations you're likely to drink more moderately. This is no coincidence. The situation around you can powerfully influence your drinking, particularly if you are unaware of its influence. Although Kirk's example may be an extreme one, triggers like those in his situation are present and operating every time you have a drink. Among the things that may influence how much you drink are:

The people you are with
The place where you are drinking
The time of day and day of the week

Hunger and thirst
How much money or alcohol is available
What you're doing besides drinking
How you're feeling

Chances are not all of these are triggers for your drinking, but some probably are. How can you find out which factors influence your drinking habits? You could just think it over, but there is a more reliable way.

In Chapter 5 we explained the self-monitoring method for keeping track of your drinking. You may remember that on the sample daily record card there was a column for "Situation." Now it's time to make use of that space.

The "Situation" column is for making notes about possible triggers, the factors that will be discussed in the following chapters. You could, for example, write down where you are whenever you record a drink. If you did, you might have some entries like those found on the record card below.

If you keep records like these for a few weeks, you may begin to notice patterns. You might observe that you were in certain places when you drank heavily (possibly at home alone or in certain bars). You might also observe that when you were in certain other places you drank more moderately. This is how your daily record cards can help you discover some triggers for your drinking.

Once you discover them, what can you do about them? That's what the next five chapters are about. They discuss five different kinds of triggers.

Sample Daily Record Card

Date	Time	Type of drink	Amount	Situation
2/20	8:30	Screwdriver	1	The pub
2/20	9:30	Bourbon	1 oz	Restaurant
2/20	9:40	Bourbon	1 oz	"
2/20	10:30	Wine (white)	6 oz	Fran's house
2/21	12:30	Bourbon	1	Home

You can use your daily record cards to find out which of these factors are most important to you. Here's how:

1. Start out by recording only one or two factors—for example, whom you're with and where you are.

2. Keep records of every drink you have and make these notes in the "Situation" column of your cards. Try this for 2 weeks or so.

3. Sit down with the cards you've kept. Lay them out and look them over, looking particularly for days when you drank more. Were you in certain places or with certain people at those times? Do you see any patterns?

4. As you become accustomed to recording the situation, add another aspect that you think might be important. What are your hunches about situations in which you overdrink? Might it be how you're feeling? What else you're doing? As you continue keeping records, see if your hunches are confirmed.

5. Don't throw your cards away. Keep them, at least until you have a clear picture of the things that may trigger your drinking or over-drinking. If you're not a regular drinker, you may have to keep records over a longer span of time to see a pattern.

Use your daily record cards to find out which kinds of triggers are most important for you.

Each of the following five chapters presents a certain kind of trigger, explaining how it can influence drinking and suggesting ways in which you can use it to cut down. As you read each chapter, consider whether the factor described may be important in your own drinking.

12

•

Places

Have you ever noticed that you tend to drink more or faster in certain places? It often happens that one gets in the habit of overdrinking in certain surroundings. The particular setting—the room, the lighting, the sounds—becomes subconsciously associated with alcohol. In a way it's like going back to visit old friends, perhaps your high school friends. You tend to act with old friends as you did when you knew them years before. Seeing them sets off old familiar behavior patterns. So it is with drinking. Some places just seem to set off overdrinking.

You may also notice that there are places in which you tend to drink less. Just as some situations make it more likely that you'll overdrink, other settings make it more likely that you'll maintain moderation or not drink at all.

Start keeping track of the places where you drink, using the "Situation" column of your self-monitoring cards as described in Chapter 11. If you find that certain places do influence your drinking, you can use this information to your own advantage.

Some places just seem to set off overdrinking.

It may be immediately obvious to you where your high-risk places are, but it can also be subtle. It may not be one particular place so much as places that have certain characteristics. Research has found, for example, that people are more likely to drink heavily in places where:

- The lights are turned down low.
- Certain kinds of music are played (for example, country western, with a slower beat that approximates your heart rate).
- The competition is high for sexual partners (for example, heterosexual men drink more when there are a lot of men and fewer women around).

- People go there specifically to drink (and get drunk).
- Other people are drinking heavily.

Conversely, people are likely to drink less when families are around, in well-lighted places, where people go for reasons other than drinking, in restaurants, and where there are activities that compete with drinking.

Places in Which You Tend to Overdrink

Suppose you discover one or more places (or kinds of places) in which you tend to overdrink. What then?

There are several possibilities. One option is to avoid them completely, at least for a while. Give yourself a break from these places. It doesn't necessarily mean you'll never go back. While "on vacation" from higher risk places, you might pick up some self-management methods from this book to help you if you do go back. Of course it's also possible that you would decide not to go back at all. People who successfully moderate their drinking often avoid their high-risk situations for a while. The same is true of people who successfully quit smoking.

If you cannot or are not willing to take a vacation from these places, you'll have to figure out ways to manage your drinking while you're there. Think of it as walking more carefully when you know you're on ice or a wet floor. Extra caution is called for when you're around your triggers. This is a particularly good time to make careful use of the methods described in Part II.

Another possibility is to change the situation somehow so you'll be more likely to exercise moderation. Here are some possibilities for breaking old habits by changing the situation.

Bars, Restaurants, or Other Public Places

If you have a favorite table or stool, move to a new one.

Take somebody along with you who will make it less likely that you'll overdrink.

Go at a different time of day or on a different day of the week.

Don't order "the usual"—have something that you're less likely to overdrink.

Take a limited amount of money with you.

At Home or Other Private Places

Change the environment around—move the furniture, change the lighting.

If there is a place where you usually sit to drink, sit somewhere else.

Change what you drink or the people with whom you drink.

Keep a limited amount of alcohol in the house.

Think creatively, "outside the box." One dad had a pattern of coming home after work and having three or four drinks before supper. It wasn't feasible for him to avoid going home, particularly because he took responsibility for watching their small children for a couple of hours while his wife went out to exercise—her first break of the day. He wanted to cut out those predinner drinks, especially after learning about BAC and how it could affect his parental responsibilities. Because he lived in a moderate climate, he decided to take the kids out to a playground after work. They liked it, and it got him out of the house and around other families, which worked well in breaking his habit of after-work drinks. Some other possibilities for him were to get a jogging stroller and go for a run with the kids; to keep no alcohol in the house and switch to thirst-quenching soft drinks; to use a flextime option to go to work 2 hours later, spending 2 morning hours with the kids (when he never drank), then working right up to supper time and thus avoiding his peak drinking hours. Usually there are several ways to change around situations that have triggered your drinking, even if you can't avoid them.

Places in Which You Tend to Drink Moderately

If you find through your record keeping that there are other situations in which you tend to drink less and maintain moderation, take advantage of this information. Spend more of your drinking time in these situations. Try to discover what it is about these situations that helps you manage your drinking.

Luke, a 34-year-old factory worker, came to our program following his second conviction for driving while intoxicated (DWI). He had written off his first DWI as "just bad luck." His second arrest had resulted in a short jail sentence and a long suspension of his driver's license. He was reluctant to seek help but decided that he needed to do something. The idea of self-management appealed to him.

Luke kept track of his drinking, including the situations in which he was drinking, for a period of 4 weeks. In looking back over his cards he found, not surprisingly, that his overdrinking episodes had taken place in the two locations where he most often drank: the Cartwheel Tavern and Loopy Lou's. He also noticed that during the month there had been nine other places in which he had drinks without going over his limit, including several restaurants, the homes of friends, and Greta's Corner. Both the Cartwheel and Loopy Lou's were dimly lit bars where men came primarily to drink. In the restaurants, on the other hand, the lighting was brighter, and there were women and children around. Greta's Corner was also a family spot, with a range of people coming and going.

Luke decided that he would go to Greta's or a restaurant or a friend's home when he felt like drinking, rather than to his two usual haunts. He decided to avoid the Cartwheel altogether, at least until he felt more comfortable in managing his drinking. Avoiding Loopy Lou's was a little harder. He had a lot of friends there, and he didn't want to take a total vacation from it. He decided that he would still go there, but not more than once a week. He also decided that when he did go, he would not go alone, because when he went alone he almost always ended up drinking too much. Rather, he would take a particular friend along and would sit at a table instead of on his usual stool at the bar. Luke hoped this would help him stick to his limits, but he made a promise to himself. If he continued to overdrink when he went to Loopy Lou's, he would stop going there altogether.

13

•

People

Just as places can affect your drinking, so can the people you're with. Certain companions may make it more likely that you'll overdrink. Heavy drinkers, for example, tend to increase the drinking rate of those around them. Obviously people who push drinks, buy rounds, ridicule moderation, or engage in drinking contests are likely to increase your alcohol consumption.

In other cases people may affect your drinking through the way you feel when you're around them. In dating situations, anxiety about impressing the other person can contribute to drinking. You may consciously or subconsciously feel a need to keep up with a companion's drinking pace. The effect can also be a kind of "reverse psychology." Feeling as if someone is trying to control or check on you, to keep you from drinking, can invite a game of hide-and-seek (I hide my drinking and you try to catch me) or just a rebellious urge to "show them."

Sometimes it's a by-product of what you do with a particular companion. If you're with someone who likes to bar-hop or party-hop, it's harder to nurse a drink slowly. Maybe you just tend to stay out later with certain companions, prolonging the period of time available for drinking.

Similarly, there are probably other companions with whom you are more likely to drink moderately, or not at all. You are probably less likely to overdrink around people who are abstainers or moderate drinkers or who support your efforts toward practicing moderation. Perhaps you drink less when you're around people with whom you feel more (or less) comfortable. How about in a room full of strangers? Again, your drinking with companions can be affected by what you usually do together. If the activities you share are ones with which drinking is usually incompatible (for example, going to a movie or going for a run), then the time you spend together is less likely to involve alcohol. With certain people (your doctor, a potential employer, a member of the clergy) you may restrain your drinking to make a more favorable impression. Thus there are also people around whom you are less likely to overdrink. Some drinkers, in fact, are most likely to overdrink when they are *away from* other people (they drink alone).

Chances are you're already thinking about the people in your life and how they may influence your drinking. A good way to find out how people affect your drinking is to use your daily record cards. Keep track of whom you are with when drinking. You can use initials to save space. After a few weeks of record keeping, examine your cards. Are there people with whom you tend to overdrink? Are there people with whom you're more likely to drink in moderation or not drink at all? What about when you drink alone? What happens when you're in a large group?

People with Whom You Tend to Overdrink

What can you do if you find you tend to overdrink when with certain people? One possibility, again, is to take a vacation from these people, to avoid them for a while. If you think you can't do that, you need to find ways of bolstering your self-control when you're around them. What is it that causes you to drink more around these people? If they push drinks on you, perhaps you need to strengthen your ability to refuse drinks (Chapter 8). If it's that they drink a lot themselves, be careful not to keep pace or compete with them. (Try having one drink to their two or stick with clock watching to pace your own drinking.) Perhaps you could meet them at places other than where you usually drink.

When you find you tend to overdrink with certain people, one possibility is to take a vacation from them.

It happens sometimes that the people you drink the most with are also the ones with whom you live or spend the most time. Some relationships turn out to be based on drinking together more than you ever realized, and changing your drinking routine can really threaten the continuation of a friendship, a business association, even a marriage. For example, it's extra hard to quit smoking when the person you live with continues to smoke. Your own efforts to reduce your drinking may be threatening to some companions because it causes them to think and wonder about their own drinking. These are tough situations, but you do have several options.

1. First, try out cutting down your own drinking and see what happens. Sometimes a companion's drinking also decreases. We treated one man who always drank with the same four friends, every night, in the same bar. He was open with his friends about what he was doing and why, and one by one they each borrowed his book and worked on their own drinking. Eventually they stopped getting together to drink. "Don't ever tell that bartender you're the one who wrote that book," he said. "You ruined his business!"

2. Second, ask for support. This requires letting your companion(s) know that you're working on managing your drinking and asking them to help you. You can add that "I'm not saying you have to change anything. I just think it's time for me to cut down, and I'd appreciate your support." Be specific about what you would like them to do (and not do) to help you achieve your goals.

3. Another possibility is to stay in contact but spend your time together in settings and activities that don't involve drinking. The underlying message here might be "I love you, and I want to be with you; I just don't want to spend our time drinking." Or "I really value you as a friend, and I want to spend time together, but I want it to be in places where I'm not so tempted to drink."

4. Then there is the difficult case in which there seems to be no way to be with a particular person without both of you overdrinking. Here you may be choosing between a relationship and your own health and happiness. It is in this situation that you may choose to take a vacation from the relationship so as to change your drinking. In the long run the relationship may be lost, but it may also be regained and strengthened. In either event, you've done what you need to do for your own health and well-being.

People with Whom You Tend to Drink Less

Whose company makes it easier for you to drink moderately? Some people find they're less likely to overdrink when in a larger group, especially if there is a good mix of men and women (or families) in the group. (Shy people, however, may drink more in larger groups.) Often, being around people of different ages inhibits one's drinking. In general, being around people who do not overdrink and who do not pressure you to drink will make it easier for you to practice moderation. Try to spend more time with the people who make it easier for you, and take them along to difficult situations. Revisit relationships that you may have neglected for a while. Try out some new friendships and groups who make it easier for you to avoid overdrinking.

Miriam was a 33-year-old university secretary who came to the self-management program after a series of embarrassing social incidents related to drinking. She wanted to learn how to drink without losing control of her behavior and judgment or taking foolish risks.

As part of her program she kept records of her drinking companions for 3 weeks. It was obvious to her, in looking at the cards, that other people did influence her drinking. When she went out with either her husband, Joe, or her friend Diana, she was likely to overdrink. When she was in larger groups and mixed company, she tended to drink less. When she drank at home alone, she almost always drank too much.

Miriam decided something had to change. She decided first of all that she would not drink alone but would always seek out friends when she was going to drink. She also resolved to take a vacation from her hard-drinking friend Diana. She decided that she would be willing to see Diana in situations in which there was no alcohol, but drinking with her would be completely out. Determining what to do about Joe was harder. Over the years she had thought several times about leaving him, but they had been together for a long time, and she really did love him. She made up her mind, though, that she would not go out drinking with him, at least until she felt more in control of her own drinking. It was when they went out drinking together that she drank most heavily. She was completely open with him about what she needed to do and why. Joe protested at first but then said that he could find "other people" to drink with. This scared Miriam, but she stuck to her commitment. As it turned out, Joe started staying home with her more often, and they also went out more often to movies and restaurants. After a few months she agreed to go out drinking with him, but only in the company of a mixed group of friends. Both she and Joe drank less on these occasions than they had before.

14

●

Days and Times

Another factor that can affect your drinking is time. Most people who overdrink are more likely to do so on certain days or at certain times of the day. Weekends, nights, paydays, holidays, and certain occasions (such as parties, football games on TV, or time in the house alone) may involve heavier drinking. Biological cycles can also affect your drinking. How fast a person metabolizes alcohol can vary with the time of day. Some people are more likely to drink when they feel tired. Drinking also fluctuates with women's menstrual cycles. The relationship of drinking to these cycles is not consistent across individuals, but it's definitely worth paying attention to as you track your own drinking.

Because you're already writing the date and time on your daily record cards, this chapter does not require any extra notes. After you've kept cards for several weeks, look back over them. Are there certain hours of the day

Paydays and Fridays are common days for overdrinking.
when you drink and others when you don't? Are there certain days of the week or month when you tend to overdrink? (Payday is a common one. So is Friday.) Are there "peak" hours or days when you tend to overdrink?

Time of Day

Sometimes people drink more heavily during certain hours. Late-night hours are often the heaviest drinking times. People who stay up later tend to drink more, and vice versa. "Morning people" (early to bed and early to rise) are less likely to overdrink than those who come alive when the sun goes down.

One common way to constrain your drinking is to impose firm time limits on it. Some people decide never to drink before a certain time or after a certain hour. One woman, for example, cut out her drinks before dinner and decided never to drink after 10 o'clock at night. If you drink in public and plan to stop at a given time, it may be easiest just to leave the drinking situation, although you could switch to soft drinks at the appointed hour. You might arrange to be interrupted by setting an appointment, receiving a phone call or text message, or having a friend pick you up.

If you restrict your drinking to certain hours, of course, it's important not to speed up your drinking at the same time. Drinking more in a shorter period of time is a recipe for high BAC. Try combining hour limits with methods for slowing down your drinking (Chapter 7) and you will have a winning combination. Drink less per hour and for fewer hours.

Drinking less per hour and for fewer hours is a winning combination for moderation.

Day of the Week

Some people drink more on weekends (or days off) than on weekdays. You might say, "Well, of course! On weekdays I have to work the next morning, so I don't drink as much." But that in itself shows that you're making conscious choices about when to drink more and when to drink less.

Sometimes people consciously or subconsciously make a decision to get drunk on certain days or nights. Again, it's a choice; if you decide to drink more on certain days, you can also decide to drink less. Some people choose to drink more on weekends. For some, Wednesday is "hump day" past the middle of the week and a drinking occasion. When you consciously decide to drink more on a certain day, it's your decision. And when you make a decision, you can plan a bit. Even if you want to feel "high," that isn't the same thing as abandoning all limits. Plan to level off before you reach your absolute limit. Arrange some controls for yourself, such as a ride home at a certain time or a limited supply of alcohol or money. These kinds of controls can be especially useful on days when natural limits (such as having to go to work) are not in effect.

Special occasions (such as weddings, holidays, religious and ethnic celebrations) are particularly risky for many problem drinkers. All of the dangers mentioned for weekends are there, plus a general atmosphere of celebration. There may be the added incentive of free drinks. When there is an open bar, people tend to drink far more than when they must purchase their own drinks. Special occasions call for special controls.

One special day that can end in overdrinking is payday, especially if it comes right before some days off. Because the availability of money is usually a factor here, a few simple preventive measures may help. Arrange to have your earnings deposited directly to your bank or deposit them yourself that day. If you do drink on higher risk days such as this, use some additional methods to limit your drinking (time limits, slower drinking, and so forth).

> It was clear to Nate, a 55-year-old furniture delivery driver, that his drinking was strongly related to time. His daily record cards showed that he tended to overdrink on weekend nights, especially between 10:00 P.M. and 2:00 A.M. Paydays (which came every other Friday) were especially heavy drinking days and were usually followed by a fight with his wife about how much money he had spent.
>
> Nate decided the best strategy would be to cut down on the hours of his drinking. He made an agreement with himself that he could drink alone on either Friday or Saturday night but not both. On the nights when he did go out alone, he arranged to stop drinking by midnight, rather than closing up the place, and to be picked up by a friend who was a taxi driver. He also planned how to make his drinks last longer so that the waitress in his favorite pub would not be pressuring him to order fresh drinks so often. Nate's agreement did allow for drinking on other nights, but only with his wife. He decided that drinking on paydays would be just too hard to control and that he would not go out alone on those nights.
>
> This plan worked fairly well. He did leave the pub by midnight on most nights out, although one night his friend forgot to come, and Nate stayed until closing time. He found, however, that moderating his drinking even before midnight was much harder in his favorite pub with the same friends. After several difficult nights, he decided to try new places. Nate also confided that he was starting to enjoy being with his wife more often.

15

•

Feelings

Finally, overdrinking often follows certain kinds of feelings. Some feelings seem to trigger drinking. Again, this is a very individual matter. A few common examples follow.

Anxiety and Stress

Alcohol, as a drug, can provide temporary relief from anxiety and physical distress. Some people drink when they become nervous or anxious, using alcohol as a relaxant or escape. Some people use alcohol as a medication to alleviate pain. Some people do find that drinking relaxes them, but there are a few things you should know about alcohol and stress.

1. Alcohol does not always relieve tension. The actual effects of alcohol on tension are complicated, but it is clear that alcohol is actually a rather poor tension- or anxiety-reducing medication for most people most of the time. Why, then, do so many people say that they drink to relax? At best alcohol sedates you to be less aware of or forget about anxiety or pain for a while, but those things are still there to greet you when your BAC level goes back down.

2. Another reason that people associate drinking with relaxation is actually superstitious. They drink at times when they would be relaxing anyhow and then give the credit to alcohol. For example, some people have a drink after a hard day. As they sit in a comfortable chair in a dimly lit room with the cares of the day behind them, they find they are, in fact, relaxing. This would probably happen with or without alcohol, at least to some extent. When alcohol is used at such times, it becomes associated with relief, and drinking increases.

WHAT WOULD YOU GUESS?

Imagine a study in which college students could drink as much as necessary to rate the taste of three different wines using a long list of adjectives.
While waiting, some of the participants were provoked to anger, insulted
by another student who was apparently also waiting to be in a study. Of
these who were angered, half had an opportunity to retaliate against the
insulting student by delivering electric shocks as part of another experiment. The other half had no opportunity for revenge. A third group was
not provoked at all, but just chatted with the waiting student. After that,
they sat down to do the wine-tasting study. Which group would you predict drank the most:

_____ Provoked to anger with opportunity to retaliate
_____ Provoked to anger with no opportunity to retaliate
_____ Not provoked to anger

The answer appears on page 117.

3. Relaxation may have little to do with alcohol itself. Researchers at
the University of Washington threw parties for students of drinking age.
College men and women gathered in a comfortable lounge, where free beer
was served. When the party was well along and the socializing noise level
was high, the host announced that there had not, in fact, been any alcohol
in the beer. The students were amazed, because they had felt pleasantly
high and very relaxed, just as if they had been drinking. If people are given
what they *believe* to be alcoholic drinks but that in fact contain no alcohol,
they still tend to relax and loosen up.[18]

4. Whatever sense of relief or relaxation comes with drinking is provided by the first few drinks. Studies have shown that when people have
more than a few drinks (getting over that 55 mg% BAC level), they actually tend to experience more negative emotions, more anxiety, or more
depression (see Chapter 4). (It's called happy *hour* for a reason!) But then
when they are sober once again, they say that they felt *better* while drinking! The trouble is that you're less likely to remember effects that occur at
higher BAC levels. It also takes time for alcohol to take effect. If you drink
rapidly, the effects of the first drinks will occur as you're having the later
drinks, leading you to believe that drinking a lot relaxes you. If you do
choose to drink to relax, drink slowly and wait for the effect to reach you.

Better still, have a look at the methods in Part IV for ideas about how to feel better without relying on alcohol.

Some people find that alcohol provides temporary release from chronic pain. Although alcohol can ease pain, again it's not a very good pain medication, and large doses can also create serious problems when used on a regular basis (see Appendix A). If your drinking is related to physical pain, consult your doctor. Describe your discomfort to him or her and explain that you've been using alcohol to relieve it. Indicate that you want to cut down on your drinking and that you would like to find an alternative means for coping with the pain. There are some very good methods to manage pain that don't involve medication.

Frustration and Anger

When something gets in your way, preventing the accomplishment of a goal, the resulting emotion is frustration. Some people drink when they become frustrated or angry. Drinking seems to be an alternative to

---

ALCOHOL FACTS: FEELING AND DRINKING

People greatly underestimate the extent to which their choices and behavior are influenced by situational factors of which they are not consciously aware.[a] Studies have demonstrated that people's drinking can be unconsciously increased by cues like background music and by inducing certain emotions. Increases in anxiety, sexual arousal, anger, or frustration can trigger heavier drinking. Anger is a common trigger for drinking, particularly in men.[b] In the study mentioned earlier ("What Would You Guess?"), men who were provoked to anger with no opportunity to retaliate (anger plus frustration) were the ones who drank the most.[c]

[a]Kahneman, D. (2011). *Thinking, fast and slow*. New York: Farrar, Straus & Giroux.

[b]Zywiak, W. H., Connors, G. J., Maisto, S. A., et al. (1996). Relapse research and the Reasons for Drinking Questionnaire: A factor analysis of Marlatt's relapse taxonomy. *Addiction, 91*(Suppl.), S121–S130.

[c]Marlatt, G. A., Kosturn, C. F., & Lang, A. R. (1975). Provocation to anger and opportunity for retaliation as determinants of alcohol consumption in social drinkers. *Journal of Abnormal Psychology, 84*, 652–659.

expressing these feelings. (In the same way, expressing these feelings seems to be an alternative to drinking; see Chapter 26.)

Depression and Disappointment

Other feelings that are often related to overdrinking are sadness, disappointment, and depression. When people experience a major loss, such as a divorce, drinking can escalate. Some people drink when they feel down, in an attempt to feel better. Disappointments in daily life are also sometimes met with an attempt to drown them in alcohol. Drinking in response to feeling down is more common in women than in men.

The problem here is that alcohol is a terrible choice as an antidepressant. In fact, alcohol has the opposite effect on the body: it is a depressant, a downer drug. Overdrinking actually increases depression and does nothing to correct its cause (see Chapters 21 and 22). It can create the illusion of helping, however, because people are less likely to remember how they felt after several drinks.

Conflict

Another common trigger for overdrinking is conflict. People sometimes drink after having an argument with a spouse, employer, or friend. Here alcohol is used as a temporary means of escaping from and forgetting the unpleasant feelings, perhaps lingering guilt or pain or anger. A better alternative here is to strengthen your skills for expressing and communicating your feelings (see Chapters 26 and 27).

You may discover that your own drinking is related to these or other feelings. One way of finding out is to keep track of your emotions on your daily record cards or in a separate diary. It's especially useful to write down how you were feeling just before you started drinking.

Sarah, a medical student, found herself drinking excessively with her fellow students in the evening after making rounds with a particularly demanding doctor, who always seemed to humiliate her in front of her peers. Her classmate Ned tended to drink too much the night before rounds were scheduled with this doctor, in the hope of calming the nerves he felt in anticipation of the stressful event. Connie overdrank whenever she started worrying about her health—which was fairly often. Her husband, Kent, drank too much after he and Connie had argued over his belief that she should be more concerned about where their kids were spending their time and less about every little physical complaint. Their oldest son, Josh, thought their home life was hopelessly depressing and had started to sneak cans of beer from the family room refrigerator up to his room.

If an emotional experience is triggering overdrinking, there are several general things that you can do:

1. You can make a commitment to yourself not to drink when you feel this way. If, for example, you find that you usually overdrink after having an argument with someone close to you, make it a point never to drink after such an argument. One common bit of advice is not to drink when you feel hungry, angry, lonely, or tired (which can be remembered through the mnemonic HALT).

Don't drink when hungry, angry, lonely, or tired; remember HALT.

2. This immediately raises the need to have some other way to respond, besides drinking, when you experience your feeling trigger. Don't just plan not to drink (that is, to do nothing). Instead, plan ahead of time what you could do instead of drinking. That's the purpose of Part IV of this book. Another general tip: when you are in a feeling-trigger situation, take extra precautions if you do drink, drawing on the methods in Part II.

3. Finally, if you're up against an emotional difficulty that just doesn't get better, consider getting some psychological consultation. Drinking almost never fixes emotional problems, and often it makes them worse. There are highly effective treatment methods available for dealing with anxiety, depression, anger, and the like.

16

Other Triggers

There are many other factors that can influence drinking. Every individual has his or her own personal pattern. We've seen people for whom the following were strong triggers for drinking:

- Reminders of a past (but unresolved) traumatic event
- The experience of being rejected or left out
- Alcohol advertisements on television
- Physical sensations that were interpreted (incorrectly) as withdrawal
- A peculiar feeling of emptiness inside
- Needing creative ideas
- Being told "No"
- Feeling powerless or helpless

Some people drink to enhance sexual experiences and have difficulty feeling aroused or disinhibited without alcohol. Beyond a drink or two, the actual physiological effect of ethyl alcohol is depressant, suppressing sexual response, and most of the aphrodisiac effect of drinking is psychological. In one study, the most sexually aroused people were those who *thought* that they had consumed alcohol but actually had been given drinks that were free of alcohol and its depressant effects.

The point is that there are many different possible triggers for drinking, some of them quite specific to individuals. In this chapter we offer just a few more common examples of the kinds of factors that can inadvertently promote overdrinking.

Thirst

Alcoholic beverages are sometimes advertised and used as thirst quench-ers. Beer in particular is promoted with this theme. From a marketing perspective it makes sense: convincing people to drink a certain product when they are thirsty would predispose them to drink more of it. If you're a person trying to manage your drinking, however, it's not a particularly good idea to drink alcohol when you're thirsty.

There is absolutely nothing better to satisfy thirst than water. From a physiological viewpoint, thirst is the body's need for water (not alcohol). Anything less than 100% water is less than 100% thirst satisfying. As a matter of fact, alcohol has a dehydrating effect. It sends blood to the periphery of your body, making your skin feel warmer (even though, in fact, you're losing body heat) and increasing sweating. Alcohol also stimu-lates the body to produce extra urine and so to lose more of its water. The superior "thirst-quenching" effect of a favorite beverage is a function of learning, imagination, and advertising and not of physiology.

Here are some tips to help you prevent overdrinking when thirsty:

1. Drink a few glasses of water or other alcohol-free beverages first. This will relieve your thirst, and you will not be using alcoholic beverages to get water into your body. This is especially important when you're dehydrated, as on a hot day or after hard work.
2. When you do drink alcohol, alternate between beverages with and without alcohol.
3. Watch out for salty foods. There is a good reason that bars provide free salty and spicy snacks: to increase your thirst.

Remember that whenever you feel thirsty, what your body really needs is water.

Hunger

Some people also overdrink when they're hungry. Alcohol does provide a quick burst of energy in the form of empty calories that contain no nutri-tion. A little alcohol can be an aperitif to whet your appetite, but the calories that come with more drinks tend to diminish hunger, leaving you drinking instead of eating healthy food. When you're hungry, try eating something first. It's always a good idea to avoid drinking on an empty stomach, both because the alcohol will hit you harder and because it can cause you to lose your natural appetite by filling you up with empty (but still fattening) calories. The alcohol alone in one standard drink provides about 100 calories, and other ingredients may add another 50 calories or more. When you feel hungry, what your body needs is nutrition.

Smoking

If you're a smoker, you probably already know that smoking and drinking can be tied strongly to each other. Puffs and sips are paired tens of thousands of times and become triggers for each other. Some have believed that you shouldn't try to give up more than one thing at a time, but research now indicates the opposite. Quitting smoking can make it easier to quit or cut down on your drinking. Stopping drinking rarely increases smoking, and stopping smoking rarely increases drinking. So if you're also thinking about quitting smoking, don't hesitate to get it over with at the same time you're working on your drinking.

Inactivity

Many people are less likely to drink when they're active. If they're involved in doing something, they tend to drink less or not at all. Heavier drinking may come with being inactive or bored. Passive pursuits, such as watching television, can also be linked to drinking more. For such individuals, it helps to stay mentally and/or physically active and particularly to do things that are not associated with drinking.

> Olive was a fascinating woman. At 60 she was a popular newspaper columnist and an active social organizer. She had no idea how or why it had happened, but she knew that her drinking was getting out of control. At times it threatened her reputation and career.
>
> Suspecting that what she did while drinking might be important, she started keeping track of her doings on her daily record cards. After several weeks she began to see a pattern. She tended to drink less when she was engaged in interesting conversation, when she was moving a lot, when she was writing, and when she played cards with her friends. She tended

to drink more when she was with people who didn't talk much, when she was watching television, when she was trying to come up with ideas for her column, and whenever she smoked. She decided that the critical factor seemed to be active engagement in something. When she was moving, working, or talking, she drank less. When she was just sitting, she tended to smoke and drink more. She had thought that drinking helped her come up with creative ideas for her column, but she found that she worked at least as well without alcohol.

Olive chose to limit her activities that were linked to overdrinking. She decided she would never drink while watching television, listening to the radio, or working. She was particularly careful to time her drinks when she was with people who were not talkative. Her occasional smoking served as a warning sign to her that she was getting bored and needed to watch her drinking more closely.

Particular Activities

For other people, overdrinking is not linked to inactivity but rather to doing *particular* things. One man we treated tended to drink more when he was in social situations in which he had to carry on a conversation. It turned out that he was painfully shy. It wasn't so much that he didn't know how to talk to people—rather, he just felt terribly self-conscious when required to do so, and this got in the way of his using his normal social skills. For some people alcohol does indeed dampen self-awareness, and that was a primary motivation for this man's heavier drinking.

In other cases, overdrinking has to do with distraction. When engaged in an activity that takes concentration and at which alcohol is also present, a person may pay less attention to drinking and lose track, particularly if others are drinking heavily. That was part of Paul's problem.

Paul was a 27-year-old lumberjack in Oregon's logging industry. His complaint was that he was "caught between a rock and a hard place." Both on the job and at home he had been having problems that he knew were related to his drinking. Yet his job, as he saw it, practically required him to stop after work "for a few." He did admit to enjoying these stops, too.

Paul began keeping daily record cards and making notes of problems at home and on the job. He expected to find that when he encountered more hassles, he would drink more, but it didn't work out that way. Instead, his records indicated that his overdrinking seemed to happen mostly on Wednesdays and on weekends and that troubles at home tended to follow rather than precede his heavier drinking episodes.

The weekends were clear enough. He stayed home on weekends and drank while watching television. But Wednesdays? Wednesday was Paul's night to shoot pool, and he quickly realized how his overdrinking was being triggered in this situation. When playing pool, he gulped his drinks between shots without really thinking about it. His attention was focused on the table. Also, most games were played for drinks, and Paul was better than average at pool. It was not unusual for him to have several beers lined up on the pool table, with his buddies egging him on: "Hey, Paul, they're getting warm!"

He also discovered that overdrinking went together with other games that he enjoyed. He liked playing cards and darts, as well as Ping-Pong at a friend's house. Whenever he became engrossed in a game, he tended to drink more, especially if he was winning drinks.

Paul developed a sudden streak of generosity on Wednesdays. He gave his opponents a handicap, so that they had to buy only half a beer for each loss. He also kept track of his drinking while playing and limited himself to one beer for each half-hour. When he won extra beers, he either refused them ("That's OK, I've already got one") or gave them away to friends ("Here, you take this one before it gets warm"). One month he even had a private contest with himself to see how many drinks he could give away in one night. His personal best was nine.

Some General Tips

Whatever the situations that may trigger your drinking, here are some tips that may be helpful.

1. **Participate in activities that compete with drinking.** Certain activities, such as running, skiing, dancing, or walking are somewhat incompatible with drinking. It's harder to do both at the same time. Look for activities that can help you drink less and do more of them. (Remember never to combine drinking with potentially dangerous activities.)

2. **Fill your time.** One of the key aspects of alcohol dependence is that it takes up a lot of time. If you're trying to avoid drinking situations, don't just do nothing. Instead, try out some of the many activities that are not typically associated with drinking. For example, people seldom drink

at the movies, at church, or during activities such as laser tag, horseback riding, or square dancing. With many sports, drinking occurs only after playing, so you can enjoy the activity but skip the postgame alcohol.

3. **Keep busy.** Passive pastimes, particularly those that involve periods of sitting or waiting (such as doing the laundry, playing computer games, watching television) can trigger overdrinking. It is easy to sip and gulp without thinking about it during such activities. If this is true for you, either avoid drinking in these situations or use additional controls such as sip counting, drink spacing, and a firm rate limit.

4. **Don't use drinks as rewards.** Avoid activities in which you "win" drinks or in which alcohol is used as a reward or celebration.

17

·

Summary: Before You Drink

Throughout Part III we've been discussing things that can trigger over-drinking. There are many different kinds of triggers, only some of which apply to you. The purpose of this part has been to help you identify those triggers that *do* matter for you and that may contribute to overdrinking in your own life. You've considered the places in which you drink, the people with whom you drink, the times when you drink, what you do when you drink, and how you feel before you drink.

There are, of course, some common trigger situations that are associated with overdrinking for many people. Here are some examples:

On weekends, holidays, or vacations
After completing a day of work, a game, or some achievement
After a stressful or emotional experience
When drinks are free or the supply is large (kegs, pitchers, punch
    bowl, and so forth)
Drinking during automatic or boring activities
When drinking is paired with activities you really enjoy
Being with heavy drinkers
When thirsty or hungry
In drinking contests or when pressured to drink faster
Drinking "the usual" in the usual place

Your basic tool for discovering the triggers or accelerators of your own drinking is to use your daily record cards. In the "Situation" column you can record anything you think might be related to how much you drink. You might write down where you are, whom you are with, what you are doing, or how you are feeling. So what do you think?

Are there places in which you are more likely to overdrink?

Are there any people with whom you are more likely to overdrink?

Are there any times or days when you're more likely to overdrink?

Do you think there are any activities that make it more likely that you'll overdrink?

Do you think you overdrink when you're feeling certain ways?

Once you discover triggers, there are at least two ways to deal with them. One is to avoid particularly difficult or tempting trigger situations. Successful changers often use this avoidance strategy during the early months of their program. Are there trigger situations that it might be best for you to avoid for the time being? Which ones?

A second strategy is to take special precautions in trigger situations, to use extra measures to strengthen self-control when in those situations. When successful changers begin to encounter their trigger situations, often after having avoided them for a period of time, they tend to be especially conscientious about using the self-control methods that work best for them, such as those described in Part II. So if there's a trigger situation you can't avoid, or when you go back into one, what can you do to be careful? What are things you could do in trigger situations to best maintain self-control? Here are a few possibilities from Parts II and III:

- Have a soft drink.
- Use the clock-watching method to space my drinks.
- Stick to a regular limit of _____ drinks.
- Drink water first.
- Keep careful drink records.
- Turn down unwanted drinks.
- Ask for support.
- Use humor.
- Have a drink that you don't like as much so you drink it more slowly.
- Do something active that doesn't involve drinking.
- Take a limited amount of money.
- Go with someone who will help and support you.
- Prearrange to leave after an hour or two.
- Have something to eat.
- Have a drink with less alcohol in it.
- Add ice.

Once you've discovered your triggers, you can choose to avoid them or to take extra precautions when you can't avoid them.

- Talk to yourself.
- Change something about the usual setting—sit somewhere new, and so forth.

Finally, it's worth noting that some people don't seem to have significant triggers. Particularly as alcohol dependence progresses, drinking just becomes regular and predictable. One man we treated had built up his drinking over a period of years to 15–20 standard drinks per day and couldn't remember the last time he had abstained from alcohol for even 1 day. There were no situations in which he seemed more likely to overdrink. He *always* overdrank, regardless of the situation, and he avoided places where he couldn't drink. As discussed in Chapter 3, once overdrinking progresses to this level, the likelihood of maintaining moderation diminishes. He wisely, albeit reluctantly, decided to stop drinking altogether, and that's what we helped him do.

Part IV

•

Instead of Drinking

Part II of this book focused on things you can do when drinking, and Part III on things that happen before drinking that can affect your self-control. Part IV examines the desired effects of drinking—the effects that people sometimes seek from alcohol. These, too, are potential "causes" of drinking and overdrinking. There can be strong motivation to drink if you're in an undesirable situation and believe that alcohol will improve matters. In essence, people sometimes use alcohol as a vehicle to get from one (less desirable) situation to another (more desirable) situation. For example, as we discussed in Chapter 15, if you're feeling depressed or anxious and you've used alcohol to feel better in the past, you're likely to do so again. If alcohol is the only way you know to change the situation, then you are dependent on alcohol to do so. So as not to rely on alcohol, you need other ways, new roads for getting where you want to be.[19]

Some people also drink because of the consequences of *not* drinking. The most obvious example of this is physical dependence on alcohol. When someone drinks large amounts over a period of time, his or her body becomes accustomed to having a certain amount of alcohol in the bloodstream. If the person stops or decreases drinking, a physical reaction occurs. This withdrawal reaction can range from relatively mild feelings of anxiety, weakness, or shakiness to severe reactions such as hallucinations and convulsions. A person who begins to experience withdrawal symptoms may drink to avoid them. Such a person is said to be *physically* dependent on alcohol and requires medical care.

There can be many other effects of not drinking. Alcohol is one way to cope with life problems, though usually not a very effective one. If it's the only way that you have to cope with certain situations, then you are *psychologically* dependent on alcohol. Psychological dependence can range from a relatively minor need, such as requiring a drink to feel like dancing, to rather major needs, such as drinking throughout the day to reduce emotional pain or anxiousness.

If alcohol is your only way to cope with a problem or meet a need, you have no choice about drinking—you must drink if that need is going to be met. If, on the other hand, you have several ways of meeting a need, one of which is alcohol, you have a choice about whether or not to drink.

Part IV illustrates alternative ways to obtain many of the effects that people seek from drinking. We think of these alternatives as personal abilities, learnable skills. These abilities are useful in meeting a variety of human needs. The more abilities you develop, the wider the range of choices you will have when deciding how to meet your needs. The wider your choice, the less dependent you are on any one solution and the freer you are to decide how you will act and feel.

Remember that six out of 10 adults are nondrinkers or drink only occasionally (see Chapter 4). They face the same challenges, joys, and sorrows that other people do. Because they choose not to use alcohol, they have learned other ways to manage their good and difficult times. You can too.

Personal Abilities

There is no exact substitute for alcoholic beverages. If what you want is to experience the precise taste and overall drug effects of alcohol, then drinking is the only way to go. Many of the effects that people desire from alcohol, however, can be achieved in various other ways. The abilities described in the following chapters represent alternative ways of producing the effects people often seek through drinking. The person who has alternatives does not need alcohol but is free to choose whether or not to drink on any given occasion.

Each of the chapters in Part IV is designed as a self-contained unit. Each one may be read individually, and they need not be read together or in order. To get the most out of these chapters, take a moment now to think about the times when you are most likely to drink (or to want a drink). What effects of alcohol are most important to you? The triggers of your drinking (Part III) may provide some clues. For example, if your drinking has often occurred when you were feeling tense, perhaps you've been using alcohol to relax, and you should read Chapter 18.

To help you decide which chapters to read first, here is a list of situations in which people often overdrink. Beside each item on the list, write an *A* next to those situations in which you have often used alcohol, a *B* next to those situations in which you have sometimes used alcohol, and a *C* next to those situations in which you seldom or never drink.

_____ At the end of (or during) a tense day (Chapter 18)
_____ When you feel out of control (Chapter 24)
_____ When faced with something you fear or are anxious about (Chapters 18 and 25)
_____ When feeling sad or depressed (Chapter 21)
_____ When you feel bad about yourself (Chapters 22 and 24)
_____ When you feel frustrated or unable to express yourself (Chapter 26)
_____ When you think you've been taken advantage of (Chapters 24 and 26)
_____ When you're not communicating well in a relationship (Chapter 27)
_____ When you are uncomfortable in a social situation (Chapters 18, 25, and 27)
_____ When you wish you were a different person (Chapter 28)
_____ When you are bored or not having much fun in life (Chapter 20)
_____ When you feel stuck (Chapter 19)
_____ When you are feeling desperate because you are not reaching your goals (Chapter 24)
_____ When you feel discouraged or demoralized (Chapters 21 and 24)
_____ When you're having problems with sleeping or getting to sleep (Chapter 23)
_____ When you feel restless (Chapters 19, 20, and 28)
_____ When you feel resentful (Chapters 19, 24, 26, and 27)

A chapters: Find the items that you have marked with an *A* and make a note of them. These are chapters to read and focus on first. Read them in whatever order you think is best. Start with the chapter that seems most important to you and find out what things you could put into practice in your life.

B chapters: You may want to read your B chapters at least once and try out the ideas presented in them.

C chapters: From your self-rating, the chapters you've labeled C are probably less important to your drinking style than the A and B chapters. Review them if you wish, after you've read the others. You may find some ideas in these chapters that are worth using in other areas of your life, whether or not they are connected with your drinking.

Needless to say, these chapters don't contain all the answers to life's problems. They do contain some ideas that have worked well for others, and whenever possible they are based on solid clinical research. See if they make sense to you and try them out. Don't make the mistake of deciding that something won't work for you before you've given it a chance. You'll never know unless you try.

Here's a helpful way to think about this: drinking alcohol is something you've practiced hundreds or even thousands of times. To replace drinking with alternative responses, you'll need to practice the new responses repeatedly before they feel as natural as drinking. This can take a while. Be persistent.

Above all, look at Part IV as a source of ideas, of possible new ways for dealing with life. You may find it helpful to browse through these chapters from time to time to remind yourself that there are many ways of getting the same results that people sometimes seek from alcohol. In the last analysis this is what matters: that you are free to meet your own needs and goals without having to depend on alcohol. We hope you'll find some of the ideas in the chapters that follow helpful to you in achieving this freedom.

A Helpful Concept: The Healthy Management of Personal Reality

As you think about things you could do to attain the same objectives you currently attain with the help of alcohol, the following image might be useful:

People respond to the day-to-day events in their lives in two main ways: by thinking about them and by doing something. Your thoughts and behaviors are what shape your personal reality, that is, your life. There are ways to react to life that produce more desirable results than others. At each moment, you can choose a response that improves your mental and emotional state, leaves it as is, or worsens it. If you're unaware that you have these choices, then you're at the mercy of chance events and responses. Once you become aware that you have some choice about the paths your thoughts and actions will take, you can begin to exert purposeful influence on your life. You can begin to shape your life and manage your personal reality. This process of "reality management" can be learned and applied to many issues in your life.

Your Internal World

Your personal reality is composed of two large elements: your *internal* world, that is, your mental world, and your *external* world, that is, the physical parts of your reality. Your internal world is made up of your thoughts and feelings (which come in many varieties), your expectations and beliefs, your memories, your goals, your self-image, and so on. We all carry on a kind of personal conversation with ourselves, which is sometimes referred to as *stream of consciousness, self-talk, chains of thought, associations,* and so on. Because these thoughts are so constant and numerous, you will often be unaware of their presence in your mind or of their impact on your emotions and actions. But, just as a persistent drop of water can eventually carve a stone, certain types of thought can eventually create an internal reality that may not be the healthiest for you. Just as a physical environment can be damaged by pollution, so can your internal environment, your mind, be harmed by toxic mental events: thoughts, destructive self-talk, lowered expectations, and mentally giving up on yourself.

At the same time, you can use thoughts to help you reach your goals, improve your emotional state, increase your positive contacts with other people, and realize that you can achieve what you choose to accomplish. Thoughts can be used to solve problems, to reward yourself, to generate alternatives, to imagine better ways of living. You can shape your internal reality to help change your personal reality. Ideas for doing this are presented throughout Part IV.

Your External World

Reality is not all in your head. What happens in your social and physical environment has a major impact on your personal reality. The external world consists of anything outside your consciousness. It includes, among other things:

- Your body
- Where you live, work, and play
- The people with whom you associate
- How much money you have
- How old you are
- Whether you are a man or a woman
- Your race or ethnicity
- Your level of education

You can shape your external world to help you attain your goals. You can begin by shaping your day: how much sleep you get, when you awaken, when you get out of bed, what you do during each hour of the day, what you eat, with whom you spend time, the specific activities that you do. Throughout Part IV, we highlight strategies that can shape your external reality as well as your inner world.

The basic idea behind Part IV is to help you shape your mind and your environment to support your goal of drinking without harming your own life or the lives of others. This can involve aiming for moderation not just in drinking but in other areas of life. For more information and help on the subjects covered in Part IV, see the Resources at the back of the book.

18

•

Relaxing

John was a plumber, and a good one. His work days were full and often included conflicts with customers, contractors, or coworkers. As the day went on, his stress level increased, and he would often end the day by saying to his assistant: "Boy, I really need a drink today!" And he would, indeed, go get a drink as soon as he left the office.

Theresa had a leadership position in a large public institution. Her days were typically filled with stressful meetings in which she was faced with challenging situations and difficult decisions. She also found that tension increased throughout the day. When she began the day already stressed, even small problems would send her "over the edge." What she had learned, however, was that if she began the day as relaxed as possible, even high levels of stress remained manageable. She began to rise early enough so she did not have to hurry through her early-morning routine and would have time to practice her new relaxation skills before leaving home. She even found small spaces in the day to practice relaxation at work.

Among people who drink more heavily, the most commonly stated reason for drinking is to feel good—to relax and change mood.[20] As a central nervous system depressant, alcohol in moderate doses does indeed relax the body to some extent, as do other drugs such as tranquilizers and barbiturates. Unfortunately, nearly all of these drugs are addicting and can have undesirable or dangerous side effects when used regularly.

Most people enjoy feeling relaxed. As a general rule, feelings of tension and anxiety are unpleasant, whereas being relaxed is pleasant. This chapter explains skills you can use to lower your tension level and increase your experience of relaxation throughout your day. You can think of this as learning to balance the levels of tension and relaxation in your life, managing your personal reality with methods that will not harm your health and well-being.

No one is able to avoid stress altogether. In fact, you wouldn't want to. Some stress is good for you—the kind that motivates you to fix a problem or that comes with change that produces long-term benefits. Excitement, although it may feel good, can also be stressful. People differ widely in the amount of stress they experience and how they respond to it. If you tend to respond to tension or tight muscles with the thought "I really need a drink," this chapter can probably be helpful to you. It provides alternative, drug-free ways to produce deep feelings of relaxation.

Because of the way the nervous system works, physical tension and psychological tension are connected. The more tense you feel subjectively, the tighter your muscles tend to become. Conversely, the tighter your muscles are, the more tense you feel subjectively. If the muscles relax, psychological tension drops as well. This is one reason people enjoy a massage. Even if you are not feeling particularly tense, relaxing your muscles can produce a very pleasant sensation—a feeling of letting go, of floating, of putting down a heavy load. By relaxing your muscles, you also use less energy and thus are likely to feel less tired at the end of the day. Similarly, if you can relax mentally, your body will tend to relax as well. The mind and body work as a unit. Therefore, learning ways to relax each in turn can give you more than one way to achieve relaxation. By adding these methods to the ones you already know, including the use of alcohol, we hope you will increase your freedom to choose.

The more tense you feel, the tighter your muscles get, and the tighter your muscles are, the more emotional tension you feel.

Many people do not know how to relax intentionally. This is not an ability that is routinely taught at home or in school—at least not yet. Because this is such a useful skill, psychologists have been experimenting for decades to find efficient ways of helping people relax. One result of this research has been an easy-to-learn method called *progressive deep muscle relaxation*. This method focuses on relaxing the body, but you will notice that it helps to relax your mind as well.

Here, in brief, are the instructions. As usual, just reading the instructions won't do a thing for you. Try it! Follow the steps closely. Read all the way through once before beginning.

Progressive Deep Muscle Relaxation

When you're ready to begin, choose a quiet room and allow yourself at least 30 minutes of uninterrupted relaxation time. Sit in a comfortable chair that has a headrest. A recliner works very well. Sit or lie back so that your arms and legs are extended and the chair supports all parts of your body. You should not have to use any muscles to support yourself. Let the chair support you. Close your eyes.

The method involves first tightening and then releasing muscles throughout your body. You do this exercise twice for each set of muscles. First you create tension in the muscle group, making the muscles as tight as possible without creating any pain or cramps. This tightness is held for about 5 seconds while you concentrate on how the tension feels. Then relax the muscles, letting them become totally loose and letting the tension go completely, and pay close attention to how the muscles feel as they are relaxing. To deepen the physical relaxation even more, you can exhale as you relax the muscles. This will relax the muscles in your chest as well and will produce a more complete feeling of well-being. The relaxed stage should last about 15 seconds. Then you repeat the procedure: tense the muscle group for 5 seconds and relax the muscles for about 15 seconds, noticing the difference in feeling. After tensing and relaxing twice, move on to the next muscle group. Never tense the muscles in a way that causes pain. The point is to pay attention to how it feels for muscles to tense and then relax, noticing the difference, and become mindful that you can bring about this feeling of relaxation at will. For the first few weeks you will be using these tensing exercises to relax fully, but eventually you can learn conscious control to relax your muscles without tensing. The goal is for you to be able to increase your level of relaxation immediately, anywhere, at any time, even in the midst of tense or anxiety-producing situations.

Here is a list of the major muscle groups to be tensed, along with descriptions of how best to tense them. Try going through the muscle groups in this order. Remember to tense and relax each group twice. Then move on to the next group of muscles.

1. *Hands.* Tighten your right hand by making a fist and squeezing. Do this twice. Repeat with the left hand.
2. *Forearms and back of hands.* With your right arm resting on the chair and the back of your hand facing up, bend your hand at the wrist, pointing your fingers straight up. Study the tension this

creates in the back of your hand and forearm. Repeat. Now do it with the left hand and arm.

3. *Biceps.* Flex the large muscles in your upper arm by trying to touch your right shoulder with your right fist, tightening the biceps. Repeat. Right arm first, then left.

4. *Shoulders.* Bring both of your shoulders up, as if to touch your ears with them. Repeat.

5. *Forehead.* Wrinkle up your forehead by bringing your eyebrows up as far as they will go. Repeat.

6. *Face.* Wrinkle your nose and close your eyes tightly. Repeat.

7. *Lips.* Press your lips tightly together. Repeat.

8. *Tongue.* Push your tongue into the roof of your mouth. Repeat.

9. *Neck.* Press your head against the back of the chair. Repeat.

10. *Chest.* Take a breath that is so deep you can feel it stretch your chest muscles. Hold it. Release it slowly. Feel yourself relax as the air leaves your lungs. Repeat.

11. *Stomach.* Suck in and tighten your abdomen, as though preparing to receive a punch in the stomach. Repeat.

12. *Back.* Arch your back away from the chair. Repeat.

13. *Legs and thighs.* Lift your legs up from the chair, holding them straight out in the air. Repeat.

14. *Calves.* Point your toes back toward your chest, creating tension in your lower legs. Repeat.

15. *Feet.* Curl your toes downward, as if digging them into sand. Feel the tension in your arches. Repeat.

After having gone through all the muscle groups and having concentrated on the difference between tension and relaxation in each of them, just stay there for a while, enjoying the experience of deep relaxation. Let yourself feel very loose, very light, very much like a deflated balloon: limp and relaxed. Notice how you feel all over your body. Do a mental check of each part of your body, letting go of any tension that remains. If any part of your body seems tense, go back and repeat the tightening–relaxing exercise for that part.

Breath Exercises

Another way to enhance relaxation is through your breathing. During the progressive muscle relaxation process described above, let your breathing become slow and even by itself. As each breath leaves your body, let it carry away more and more tension and take you deeper and deeper into relaxation.

A simple exercise that you can do most anywhere is to draw in a deep breath and then release it slowly. Some people find it helpful to think of a calming word like "peace" as they release the breath. Do this at least five times, with your eyes closed if possible, and you are likely to feel tension draining away.

If you have a bit more time, try a variation called "deep sleep breathing." You can practice this for as long as you like—or until you fall asleep! The pattern here is to draw in a deep breath gently, just until the lungs feel full, and then slowly release it. There is a natural pause after you exhale, before your body naturally draws another in breath. This is the opposite of gasping—a relaxed, natural rhythm of breathing like deep sleep. Don't make any effort to draw in an extra-large breath or to lengthen the pause after you exhale. Just let it happen.

Visual Images for Relaxing

Another tip for deeper relaxation involves bringing your thoughts into harmony with your physical state. You have relaxed your muscles and breathing in order to relax your mind. You can also relax your mind to further relax your body. Certain visual images may bring your thoughts into balance with your relaxed physical state. These images can be used either by themselves or in conjunction with your relaxation practice. They are meant to deepen your relaxation.

1. **Putting down a load.** Imagine yourself carrying all your responsibilities in a big sack on your shoulders. Once you're ready to begin relaxing your muscles, as you sit quietly with your eyes closed, imagine yourself putting down your load. For the time you've allotted to do relaxation, you don't have to worry about it. You are responsible for nothing. You don't have to *do* anything but relax. You can just enjoy *being*.

2. **The marionette.** This image is particularly good to use during the time when you are tensing and relaxing your muscles. Think of a marionette standing up straight, being held up by taut strings that make it move. If the marionette operator's hands let go of the strings, they will go loose and the marionette will crumple into a totally relaxed heap. Now: Your brain is the marionette operator and can let go of you whenever it

wants to. As you relax each muscle, imagine letting go of the marionette strings, and as your body goes limp, your mind ceases to labor as well and can enjoy relaxing fully.

3. **The balloon.** Imagine yourself as a balloon that has been inflated to full capacity. It is tight, tense. As you use the breathing exercise to help you relax, imagine you're letting air escape from the balloon. As more and more air escapes, the tightness decreases, the tension disappears. You become wonderfully limp and relaxed.

4. **The cloud.** Imagine yourself as a cloud, a calm and fluffy cloud. You are floating pleasantly in the middle of a clear blue sky. Feel the wind touching your face. Feel the warmth of the sun. Feel how light you are. Enjoy the peaceful sensation.

Now stop reading for a while and conjure up one of these images. Find an image that is most relaxing for you.

What other images would be relaxing for you? Tailor them to fit you. They might be images of unwinding, letting go, floating, melting, flowing, smoothness, pleasing warmth or coolness, peacefulness, lightness, having nothing to worry about. You might use the image of a particularly beautiful and relaxing place where you have been or would like to go.

Applications

Remember, the purpose of these techniques is to help you relax more deeply. By practicing deep muscle relaxation as described once or twice a day for 2 weeks, you will noticeably increase your ability to achieve the relaxed state. Then start experimenting. Try to reach the deep state of relaxation without tensing all of your muscles. Focus on creating the "letting go" feeling that you have been observing as your muscles relax. Use the breathing techniques or relaxing images. How deeply can you relax without the tensing exercises?

When you're able to relax without the tensing exercises, you can use this relaxation almost anywhere. Take a mental inventory of your body tension during the day—perhaps at work or at lunch. This is when the methods really begin to become useful. Even after you can relax on your own, you should go through the whole tensing–relaxing procedure from time to time, just to remind yourself how deep relaxation can be.

Once you can relax without tensing, begin to apply your new skill in daily living. Start with a relatively slow activity. Try relaxing, for example, while reading the paper. Relax as completely as you can without tensing your muscles first. Draw and release some deep breaths. Allow all muscles to relax except for the ones you're using at the moment. Here are some other slow activities in which you can begin.

Watching television, a movie, or a play
Playing cards, chess, checkers, or other table games
Sitting and talking with others
Waiting in line
Riding a bus
Driving

Once you can relax during these slower activities, begin relaxing during some more demanding activities, such as:

Shopping
Doing housework
Washing the car
Having a conversation
Playing ping-pong or pool

Finally, begin using your relaxation skills during the fastest, most demanding activities you can think of:

Jogging (yes, you can relax while you run; athletes do)
Running to catch a bus
Being in a crowded place
Rushing to finish a project
Playing tennis, football, or other sports
Talking to a very angry person
Taking care of an emergency

It is possible to relax and move rapidly. Athletes and dancers are trained to remain loose as they perform. If some of your muscles are tight and tense, they will prevent other muscles from doing their jobs smoothly. In addition, you will use a lot of energy needlessly.

Many people drink to relax, but there are a number of ways to relax besides drinking.

There are other ways of achieving bodily relaxation. Some people find that yoga, meditation, tai chi, or massage helps them relax. There are often classes available on these activities. You could find out if there are any in your area and explore what participation would involve.

So what does all of this have to do with drinking? As we mentioned at the beginning of this chapter, many people drink to relax and feel better, but there are a number of ways to do this besides drinking. If you're skilled in deep muscle relaxation, yoga, meditation, or self-massage, you don't need alcohol to relax you. You have other alternatives. You will have the option of using alcohol, but it will no longer be your only option.

The next time you feel you "need" a drink to relieve stress, ask yourself what you could do instead.

One final tip relevant to drinking: When people have had a bad experience—a hard day, a harrowing time, a frustration, a scare—they sometimes have a drink. Then the stress begins to decrease, and they think, "Ah, how relaxing alcohol is!" Next time this happens to you, try doing something else to relax. No matter what you do after a stressful experience, the most likely result is that your tension will start going down. It's automatic, because people just don't maintain high levels of physical or mental stress for very long. If you started knitting immediately after each stressful experience, you would probably find knitting rather relaxing after a while. Let the tension pass first. Relax yourself. Then decide whether or not you want to drink.

These, then, are some alternative ways of dealing with stress. The next time you feel you "need" a drink to relieve stress, ask yourself what you could do instead. The more often you can successfully use another method, the more likely it is that drinking alcohol will become a real choice and not a necessity.

19

●

Self-Talk

Victor had been having trouble talking to his 17-year-old daughter. It seemed that every time they got into a conversation it turned into an argument. They ended up getting angry at each other and feeling as if they would never be able to communicate. There were things she did that really burned him up, but he also knew that he made things worse by reacting to her irritating habits as he did. Invariably these interactions ended when she stalked off in a huff. And almost every time this happened, he would head for the refrigerator to open up a can of beer. He wished he had a coach to suggest a good play to use when he was in the middle of the fray. He thought a mental "time-out" might do the trick when he started getting mad. If he continued responding in his usual knee-jerk way, things were not going to change. Even though he was often angry at his daughter, he knew he loved her and she loved him, and he wanted to do his part to improve their relationship before she left home after graduating from high school.

If you observe yourself carefully when making a difficult or even a simple choice, you will discover that a silent conversation is going on within you.

Should I wear dressy or casual clothes? Most people will probably be dressed up, but I feel more comfortable in sport clothes. Should I do what everybody else is going to do? Will it bother anybody if I dress casually? Not really. The worst that can happen is that some people will notice that I'm not as well dressed as the rest. That's no big deal. I'll go casual.

Of course this happens so fast that you usually don't pay attention to it. Often there is no need for you to do so.

What is happening, though, is a process that is very useful in guiding your actions. This process becomes more noticeable when you are faced with either a new problem or a difficult situation. It's almost as if there were a committee inside you, working out decisions. You can hear them talking most loudly when you have a tough decision to make.

You may also be aware of self-talk when learning a new skill. Someone learning tennis, for example, may silently say "Now keep your eye on the ball" and "Toss it straight up." New skiers tell themselves "Bend your knees!" The voice of the coach becomes your own. Adolescents learning to drive are (we hope and pray) silently reminding themselves to watch for traffic lights, press the pedals in a smooth motion, and watch out for pedestrians and bicycles.

Talking to yourself silently is really a fairly natural process. The purpose of this chapter is to show you how you can harness the power of this self-control strategy by using it systematically. You can learn to use self-instructions in a way that will help you carry out your plans more consistently. You can learn to be your own coach.

How does this ability fit into your program to moderate your drinking? One of the challenges you may meet as you put the methods in this book into practice is that there will be times when you are confused or uncertain about how to handle a particular situation. It may seem easier to have a drink and put the whole thing off until you feel more like tackling it.

So there you are, wishing someone was around to give you some advice or to suggest something to help you through this rough situation. There's just no one who can do that for you all the time. Or is there?

The fact is that you can do it yourself. For most of the tough situations that you have to face, chances are you probably have good ideas as to how to handle them effectively. Sometimes you can prepare yourself before the situation arises, while there is less pressure to come up with a solution. If nothing else, you can at least reassure yourself and calm yourself down so that you don't make the situation more difficult by feeling overwhelmed. Treat yourself as you would treat a friend in the same situation. Offer yourself some sound advice as though it were coming from a caring and wise friend. In a way it is probably easier for you to tailor advice for yourself because you know better than anybody else what you are feeling and what

You can learn to be your own coach. it is that you want to do.

Here are some steps for talking to yourself intelligently:

1. Make a list of common situations in which you could use a little guidance. For example:

Keeping to my limit of drinks
Being more sociable at a party
Concentrating at work
Reducing stress and tension
Others:

_____

_____

_____

2. Plan ahead. Think through the kinds of problems you usually encounter in each situation. Prepare instructions you could use to deal with each problem. It may help to think of these self-instructions as falling into two categories: ways to shape your external reality (physical, observable reality, that is, what you do) and ways to shape your internal reality (your mental reality, that is, what you think).

Here are some examples of self-instructions for how to shape your external reality (what you do physically):

Drink slowly. Take smaller sips. Order a drink containing no alcohol.
Ask someone's name. Smile when talking to somebody.
Set short deadlines for yourself. Say "Stop!" when your daydreams are
    keeping you from completing what you've chosen to do.
Check out your body for tension and relax parts that feel tight.
Let your breathing relax you. Picture relaxing scenes.

Here are some examples of self-instructions for how to shape your internal reality (what you do mentally):

Remind yourself that you can stick to your decision.
Argue in your mind against the nonsensical idea that you *have* to have
    a drink.
Dump the idea that you have to prove yourself to anybody.
Remind yourself that you are as interesting as anybody here.
Don't berate yourself about daydreaming. Just go right back to working.

Say to yourself, "I can deal with tension. I know how to relax."
Rule Number 1: Don't freak out! [Or: Don't panic!]
Write down your own useful self-instructions:

_____

_____

_____

3. Try out these self-statements as soon as you get a chance. If you don't find yourself in any of the situations you prepared for, they weren't common enough. Add others that happen more often.

4. Modify your self-coaching statements until they feel right. You may need more specific statements about what to do. You may find that as long as you remind yourself to stay calm, you handle the situation fine. Try this out and learn about yourself!

Victor wrote down "talking to daughter" as one of his problematic situations. He prepared these "what to do" instructions for this situation:

> *Don't raise your voice.*
> *Let her say what she has to say.*
> *Tell her what you think she said. Make sure you heard it right.*
> *Tell her which parts of what she said you agree with.*
> *Then tell her your opinion about the things you disagree with. Just say it; you don't have to act it out for her.*
> *And above all, don't feel that you're defeated if you don't get her to change her mind. That sets you up for failure.*

His instructions for "what to feel" were:

> *Be prepared to go from irritated to really angry.*
> *Think of it as an experiment and see if you can stop at "irritated."*
> *If it doesn't work, you're no worse off than before.*

Remind yourself that having a good relationship with her and having her do what she wants to do anyway is better than having a bad relationship with her and still having her do what she wants to do anyway. (Don't assume that if you fight with her as before she will do what you want. That has not worked so far.)

It wasn't more than 2 days before Victor found himself right in the middle of a conversation with his daughter that threatened to blow up. He began by telling himself, "OK. This is where I want to be able to handle things better." Then he began to use the instructions that he had prepared. "Keep your voice down, Vic. Listen to her." During the conversation his daughter began to work herself up as usual. When she saw that Victor was not blowing up, she seemed to quiet down a little. It was as if she had been getting ready to stand up to his anger and then found there was no need to. She didn't change her mind, but at least the conversation ended without a mishap. Victor told himself, "If you can keep on controlling your temper, you might actually start enjoying talking to her."

Victor thought over what he had done and decided there were two things he wanted to change in his instructions. One was the fact that, even though he had kept his voice down, he heard himself sounding sarcastic and preachy a couple of times. That was not a good substitute for yelling, so he added this: "Don't try to get at her by scolding, preaching, or making fun of her. You want her to stay calm, too." The second thing he had noticed was that he had rewarded himself mentally when he had followed his instructions carefully. That had seemed to help. He decided to tell himself, when he was succeeding in keeping to his plan, "Good, Vic! You did that just right. Good try! Keep it up! You're getting good at this." Being able to give himself instructions seemed to Victor to be something like having a coach at his side whenever he needed help. That in itself made him feel more hopeful.

Self-instruction can be used in combination with any of the other techniques in this book. You can remind yourself how to handle certain situations and to keep yourself focused on what it is that you want to do. Study a technique in this book—one that you really want to remember to use. Then put the technique in your own words. Prepare some instructions for yourself. Carry them with you.

Finally, self-talk can be helpful if your motivation to maintain moderation begins to wane. Begin to notice the "helpful" and "harmful" thoughts that occur to you. The helpful thoughts are those that come from a caring and wise perspective. The harmful thoughts are those that come from a resentful, rebellious, I-don't-care or I-don't-give-a-damn perspective. You'll hear someone on that internal committee we all have in our heads say, "Oh what's the use?" or "Just a few more won't hurt" or "Why can't I just drink as much as I want?" At times like this it is important to call on other members of the committee to remind you why what you are doing is important. What are the most persuasive and important reasons for you to moderate your drinking? You can, of course, drink as much as you choose, but why have you decided not to do so? Even when the alcohol-dependent committee member's voice gets loud, you don't need to let him or her take over the meeting. There are perfectly good reasons why you've chosen to drink moderately. What are they? (If you have a hard time remembering them, begin writing them down again here, so they will be ready for you to use.)

Self-instruction can be used in combination with any of the other techniques in this book.

_____

_____

_____

20

Pleasant Activities without Alcohol

Toni's company recently moved her to a new city. Although she had originally been excited about the move, she soon found that she missed a lot of her friends and, surprisingly, a lot of the places she frequented in her former city—not only the parks and malls, but even the fast-food restaurants and supermarkets. She found that instead of going out two or three evenings a week as she had done back "home," she was going out at most once a week. In addition, although at first she had been in rather frequent contact with her old friends, as the weeks went on she heard from them less and less. Her mood started sliding, and, when people she had met did call her to do something together, she often found an excuse because she just did not feel like going out. Soon they stopped calling.

What finally snapped Toni out of this vicious cycle was that she found herself drinking heavily more and more often while alone in her apartment. She had gone through a period like this before and did not want this one to last as long as the previous one had. She began systematically planning activities a couple of nights a week and at least one special activity on Sunday. She called some of the people who had called her before and invited them out. But even more important, she began to seek out new places to frequent where she felt comfortable and "at home." Though at first she had to force herself to do this, as the days went by her mood improved, and she felt more and more like going out and enjoying the new people and the new places she was discovering. Her drinking returned to its normal moderate level, in large part because she was out and about and too involved with her newfound activities to be drinking at home alone.

What You Do Affects How You Feel

Your mood and health are influenced by what you *think*. They are also powerfully influenced by what you *do*. To maintain a reasonably happy and balanced life, it is important to do things that you find pleasurable. It's a bit like taking daily vitamins. Having a good number of pleasant events scattered throughout each week is like making sure you have enough to eat and get enough sleep. In fact, human beings may have a "minimum daily requirement" of pleasant and reinforcing activities. Keeping a good balance of fun and pleasant events in your life is important to maintaining psychological health.

An important step in becoming free of alcohol dependence is to discover that pleasure and fun do not require intoxication.

What happens if your life becomes short on pleasant events and fun? One common result is a drift toward depression.[21] Ironically, when you become depressed, you feel even less like doing the things you normally find pleasant. The result is a downward spiral. (If you feel you're having problems that resemble depression, see Chapter 21.)

Happily, this spiral also works in reverse: when you build pleasurable events into your life, even (and especially) when you don't feel like doing them, your mood tends to improve. You're less likely to feel depressed when you're engaging in pleasant activities regularly. When you get to feeling down, then, one thing to ask yourself is how many pleasant events you have participated in recently and how many you have planned for the near future.

Human beings may have a "minimum daily requirement" of pleasant and reinforcing activities.

It's worth noting here that people who drink heavily often tend to equate having fun with drinking. The reason, in part, is that their pleasant times and activities have so often been accompanied by drinking. Some people say that they literally haven't had fun except when drinking. As a depressant drug, alcohol itself isn't a particularly good choice for improving mood. (Think about drinking alone, for example.) It's just that alcohol is so often paired in experience (and certainly in advertising) with having a good time. As mentioned earlier, the relaxation and loosening-up that occur in social drinking situations also occur when people think they are drinking alcohol even though they are not. An important step in becoming free of alcohol dependence is to discover that pleasure and fun do not require intoxication.

So what can you do if your life is short on pleasant activities that do not require drinking? Here are some steps:

1. *Make a reasonably long list of those things you like to do.* Some possible categories are:

Things I can do alone:

_____

_____

_____

Things I can do with one or more other people:

_____

_____

_____

Physical activities:

_____

_____

_____

Intellectual activities:

_____

_____

_____

Productive activities:

_____

_____

_____

Restful activities:

_____

_____

_____

Things that take only a few seconds:

_____

_____

_____

Things that take a couple of minutes:

_____

_____

_____

Things that require a couple of hours:

_____

_____

_____

Things that take a few days:

_____

_____

_____

Things that don't cost anything:

_____

_____

_____

Things that cost a little:

_____

_____

_____

Things that cost a lot:

_____

_____

_____

Activities at home:

_____

_____

_____

Activities in the city:

_____

_____

_____

Activities in the country:

_____

_____

_____

Make a list of specific things you can do, using these categories to suggest ideas. Be sure they are things that *you* enjoy, not just things that are supposed to be pleasant. Sometimes it's helpful to think of things that you used to enjoy doing but haven't done recently for some reason. Have you stopped going to the movies in favor of watching DVDs at home? Given up hikes in the woods? Canceled your subscription to a cooking magazine that used to inspire you to experiment with new cuisines? Quit playing tennis or touch football? Also consider things that you *might* enjoy—activities about which you've thought at times "That might be fun." There's one way to find out.

Are you having trouble coming up with ideas? Enter "pleasant events schedule" in an Internet browser for hundreds of ideas.

2. *Schedule time to do some of these things.* Planning and scheduling leisure time may seem strange to you, but think of it this way: Having rewarding leisure time is important to your mental health. It keeps you going so that you can function well in other areas of your life. Isn't it just as important to schedule leisure, then, as it is to schedule appointments, a checkup with your doctor or dentist, or regular meetings? Making Friday night "movie night" or arranging to play tennis with a friend one morning a week can ensure that you follow up on your intentions to have a good time.

3. *Make sure there's variety in your leisure activities.* Many things that are a lot of fun can lose their pleasure if done too often. This is why it's good to have a long list of possible pleasant activities: it gives you a good menu from which to choose. And doing something too often may be why you stopped pursuing a pastime that was once a favorite. If you tire of one sport, for example, is there another you might enjoy?

4. *Remind yourself that it's OK to have fun.* Fun lifts your spirits and helps you function better in other areas of your life. Recreation should be a regular part of your life. If it helps to get you back into the habit, think of it at first as a reward for all the work you do. It won't take long for you to consider fun as much a part of your routine as going to sleep at night or eating meals.

21

Coping with Negative Moods and Depression

Jerry's friends knew that when he called them and said "Let's go get drunk," he meant "I'm hurting and I need company." They worried about him when this started happening more and more often, but they had already set up a well-worn pattern in which they drank together without prying into whatever was bugging him. It wasn't until he began not showing up for work and they heard that he might be fired that they decided to break the pattern and ask him directly what was going on. He had clearly become seriously depressed and had even begun to have thoughts of suicide. They urged him to get help from the employee assistance program, which he finally agreed to do.

Over the ensuing weeks, Jerry learned other ways to deal with his depression. His friends stood by him and arranged activities so they could be with him without drinking alcohol. Once the depression cleared, they were able to go back to having a few beers. But they had learned from Jerry that the alcohol itself could be a trigger for depression in him. Because he did not want to go through the very painful experience of severe depression again, he had decided not to go over his self-chosen limit of one or two drinks per night. His new way of asking for company changed to "Let's go get a drink!" And his friends, more than happy to have him back, respected the limits he had chosen.

Perhaps you've turned to alcohol after having an argument with someone, failing at something, or being insulted or rejected. Some people drink when they're feeling down or blue. "Drowning our sorrows" has become such an accepted way of responding to hurt and disappointment that we often brush aside a truth that's undeniable to those who have ever tried it: alcohol is a depressant drug that is likely to worsen your mood in the long run and often in the short run, too.

Everyone experiences negative moods at times. Sometimes these moods turn into depression. Sometimes it's a matter of being generally "down"—lacking zest and enthusiasm without knowing why. At other times it may be in response to a specific disappointment, loss, or frustration.

Whatever the cause, you begin to slow down. Your energy level is low, and you don't feel like doing anything. If it gets bad enough, you may start to eat less or have trouble sleeping. How can you deal with this common experience?

The first step is to consider whether what you are feeling is a bothersome but common negative mood or whether it might be a serious depression. About 7% of all adults in the United States suffer from a serious depression (called a "major depression") in any one year, and 16% suffer from a serious depression at some time in their lives. Women are almost twice as likely to suffer from such a depression as men are.[22]

If you have been noticeably depressed for a while, or if you tend to drink more when you are depressed, we suggest you fill out the questionnaires on pages 157 and 158. *Complete them before reading on to our explanation of what they mean, so that your scores will not be influenced by our explanation.*

A Note on Screening Instruments

Before you score your questionnaires, it's important to understand two things about screening instruments:

1. **Screening instruments do not yield a diagnosis.** When well constructed, screening instruments inquire about the presence of symptoms that are considered to be part of the condition being assessed. For example, the two questionnaires you just filled out have to do with depression. The Mood Screener inquires about the symptoms that a professional looks for to decide whether a person is suffering from major depression. If you gave accurate answers, and if your score shows that you are not experiencing the symptoms of major depression, it is very unlikely that you have this condition. If you *are* experiencing the symptoms, it is *possible* that you are suffering from major depression, but, of course, these symptoms could be

The Mood Screener

Name: .... Date: ....

	A. Lifetime		B. Current	
	Have you ever had two weeks or more when nearly every day you...	Check if any answers were "Yes"	Have you had this problem nearly every day in the last two weeks?	Check if any answers were "Yes"
❶ Felt sad, blue, or depressed most of the day nearly every day?	❑ Yes ❑ No	1 ❑	❑ Yes ❑ No	1 ❑
❷ Lost all interest or pleasure in things you usually cared about or enjoyed?	❑ Yes ❑ No	2 ❑	❑ Yes ❑ No	2 ❑
❸ a. Lost or increased your appetite nearly every day?	❑ Yes ❑ No		❑ Yes ❑ No	
b. Lost weight without trying to? (Over 2 lbs. [1 kilo] per week)	❑ Yes ❑ No	3 ❑	❑ Yes ❑ No	3 ❑
c. Gained weight without trying to?	❑ Yes ❑ No		❑ Yes ❑ No	
❹ a. Had trouble falling asleep, staying asleep, or waking up too early?	❑ Yes ❑ No		❑ Yes ❑ No	
		4 ❑		4 ❑
b. Been sleeping too much nearly every day?	❑ Yes ❑ No		❑ Yes ❑ No	
❺ a. Talked or moved more slowly than is normal for you?	❑ Yes ❑ No		❑ Yes ❑ No	
		5 ❑		5 ❑
b. Had to be moving all the time, that is, couldn't sit still and paced up or down?	❑ Yes ❑ No		❑ Yes ❑ No	
❻ a. Felt tired or without energy all the time?	❑ Yes ❑ No	6 ❑	❑ Yes ❑ No	6 ❑
❼ a. Felt worthless, sinful, or guilty nearly every day?	❑ Yes ❑ No	7 ❑	❑ Yes ❑ No	7 ❑
❽ a. Had a lot more trouble concentrating or making decisions than is normal for you?	❑ Yes ❑ No		❑ Yes ❑ No	
		8 ❑		8 ❑
b. Noticed that your thoughts came much slower than usual or seemed mixed up nearly every day?	❑ Yes ❑ No		❑ Yes ❑ No	
❾ a. Thought a lot about death— either your own, someone else's, or death in general?	❑ Yes ❑ No		❑ Yes ❑ No	
b. Wanted to die?	❑ Yes ❑ No	9 ❑	❑ Yes ❑ No	9 ❑
c. Felt so low you thought about committing suicide?	❑ Yes ❑ No		❑ Yes ❑ No	
d. Attempted suicide?	❑ Yes ❑ No		❑ Yes ❑ No	
		Number of boxes checked: = ____		Number of boxes checked: = ____
Did these problems interfere with your life or activities a lot?	❑ Yes ❑ No	❑	❑ Yes ❑ No	❑

Source: The Mood Screener was developed by Ricardo F. Muñoz, PhD, University of California, San Francisco. Questions are adapted from the Diagnostic Interview Schedule, which is in the public domain. See Robins, L. N., Helzer, J. E., Croughan, J., et al. (1981). National Institute of Mental Health Diagnostic Interview Schedule. *Archives of General Psychiatry, 38*(4), 381–389. The Mood Screener can be reproduced without permission from the author. Reprinted in *Controlling Your Drinking* (2nd ed.).

Center for Epidemiological Studies—Depression Scale (CES-D)

Name: .... Date: .... Total score: ....

Below is a list of ways you may have felt. Please indicate how often you have felt this way during the past week: rarely or none of the time; some or a little of the time; occasionally or a moderate amount of time; or most or all of the time.

During the past week, that would be from _____ through today: (date)	Rarely or none of the time (less than 1 day)	Some or a little of the time (1–2 days)	Occasionally or a moderate amount of time (3–4 days)	Most or all of the time (5–7 days)
1. I was bothered by things that usually don't bother me.	0	1	2	3
2. I did not feel like eating; my appetite was poor.	0	1	2	3
3. I felt that I could not shake off the blues even with help from my family or friends.	0	1	2	3
4. I felt that I was just as good as other people.	3	2	1	0
5. I had trouble keeping my mind on what I was doing.	0	1	2	3
6. I felt depressed.	0	1	2	3
7. I felt that everything I did was an effort.	0	1	2	3
8. I felt hopeful about the future.	3	2	1	0
9. I thought my life had been a failure.	0	1	2	3
10. I felt fearful.	0	1	2	3
11. My sleep was restless.	0	1	2	3
12. I was happy.	3	2	1	0
13. I talked less than usual.	0	1	2	3
14. I felt lonely.	0	1	2	3
15. People were unfriendly.	0	1	2	3
16. I enjoyed life.	3	2	1	0
17. I had crying spells.	0	1	2	3
18. I felt sad.	0	1	2	3
19. I felt that people disliked me.	0	1	2	3
20. I could not get "going."	0	1	2	3

Source: This scale is in the public domain. See Radloff, L. S. (1977). The CES-D Scale: A self-report depression scale for research in the general population. Applied Psychological Measurement, 1, 384–401. Reprinted in Controlling Your Drinking (2nd ed.).

caused by a number of other conditions. This is why it is important that a professional who is trained to recognize and diagnose depression conduct a formal assessment. Only a trained professional is qualified to render a diagnosis. The questionnaire is only a tool to determine whether you have the symptoms of major depression, and, if you believe depression might be affecting your life, you should seek further evaluation.

2. **Screening instruments do not rule out the possibility that you have some other problem.** If your score on these two screening tests indicates that you do not have symptoms of depression, you might still be suffering from another problem. Diagnostic categories are merely tools to help professionals decide what type of treatment is most appropriate. If you're experiencing serious emotional pain or if your problems are interfering with your life or activities a lot, seeking help is the most reasonable step to take, no matter how you score on these two tests.

The Mood Screener

We've included the Mood Screener in this chapter because major depression is one of the most common emotional problems and is often associated with excessive drinking. Health care professionals usually inquire about nine symptoms that are considered in determining whether a person is suffering from major depression. The Mood Screener asks questions about these particular nine symptoms. The first two columns ask if you have *ever* had the major depression symptoms. The last two columns refer to whether you are having the symptoms *now* (within the past 2 weeks).

Scoring the **Mood Screener**: *If, for any of the nine numbered rows under "Lifetime," you have answered at least one "yes," you can fill in the box in the second column. Then add up the number of boxes from 1 to 9 and enter that number on the bottom row. Do the same for the last two rows, under the word "Current."*

If you marked five or more of the nine boxes in the "Current" columns, including either symptom 1 (feeling depressed) or symptom 2 (losing interest or pleasure), and marked "yes" to the question "Did these problems interfere with your life or activities a lot?" it is possible that you are currently having a period of major depression. If that is the case, we recommend that you see your primary-care physician, show her or him the list of symptoms you're having, and ask whether your feelings of depression warrant either treatment or a referral to a specialist on depression.

Your primary-care physician can prescribe antidepressant medication or can refer you to a psychologist, psychiatrist, social worker, or other mental health specialist.

If you marked five or more of the nine boxes in the "Lifetime" columns, *and* you also answered "yes" to the question "Did these problems interfere with your life or activities a lot?" you may have had a period of major depression sometime in the past. However, if you don't have these symptoms currently, you probably are not in the middle of a major depressive episode at this time. In that case, we recommend that you move forward with your plans to moderate your drinking, but be attentive to your mood levels. People who have had a major depressive episode in the past are more likely than others to have another one. If you notice depressive symptoms increasing, go through the Mood Screener again, and, if you are experiencing five or more symptoms, seek help earlier rather than later. The longer a depressive episode lasts, the more it can affect your personal relationships, your work productivity (and reputation), and your overall ability to enjoy life. The earlier you begin to treat it, the easier it is to get back to normal quickly.

The Center for Epidemiological Studies— Depression Scale (CES-D)

What if you have not had five or more of these symptoms, but you are still feeling down? Are your negative moods within the average range of mood for adults in the United States? The second questionnaire provides some guidance here. The CES-D has been used in many large-scale community studies, and therefore there is a fair amount of information about what the scores mean. The CES-D scores are not a screener for major depression. They represent a range of depressed *mood*, from average mood levels to high levels of depressed mood. If your mood score is high, you are more likely to use alcohol, tobacco, or other drugs excessively. Therefore, your score can serve as a reminder that you need to learn to manage your mood in other ways if you want to be successful in moderating your drinking.

To score the CES-D, make sure you have answered every one of the 20 items and that you have circled only one number in each row. Then add up all the numbers you circled. Your score should be somewhere between 0 and 60. The higher the score, the stronger your feelings of depression.

Interpretation of scores:

Less than 16: clearly within the average range of scores for adults in the United States

16 to 24: borderline elevation of depressed symptoms, compared with other adults

24 and above: significant elevation of depressed symptoms, compared with others

If you scored less than 16, depressed mood does not seem to be a current issue for you. If you scored 16 to 24, depressed mood may be a source of concern for you, and it may be worthwhile for you to put the material in this chapter into practice to prevent the level of depression from getting worse.

If you scored 24 or above, you should definitely attempt to bring your level of depression down. If you did not currently have the five symptoms of major depression in the Mood Screener, it's possible that your score on the CES-D reflects a temporary period of stress. However, if this continues for long, it could eventually develop into a major depressive episode or another form of serious depression.

Note, however, that these scores vary widely depending on your position in society. For example, although the average score on the CES-D is 8.7 for people ages 25 to 74, women do tend to score higher than men. Moreover, among individuals living alone, men's average score is 8.5, and women's 10.8, whereas for people living with others, men's average score is 6.8, women's average score is 9.3, and the average for women who are heads of households is 12.5. People with less education and lower income tend to score higher.

Ways of Thinking about the Connection between Drinking, Mood, and Depression

All human beings need to learn how to regulate their own mood states as they develop. Some of us have learned to do so better than others. If you began using alcohol (or tobacco or another psychoactive substance) when you were a teenager, you may have learned to use it to deal with many of the new situations encountered during adolescence. That means that, as you reduce your use of alcohol to deal with your mood, you may need to learn new ways to keep your mood within a healthy range.

Although it's fairly common for people to drink when they feel down or depressed, alcohol actually makes matters worse. Because alcohol is itself a depressant drug, it tends to perpetuate rather than alleviate depression. Its appeal may lie in the fact that during a period of intoxication you forget your problems ("drowning your sorrows") and generally shut down, but on sobering up you inevitably find the problems are still there and your mood tends to be worse, which in turn may encourage more drinking.

Alcohol is a depressant drug, which tends to perpetuate rather than alleviate depression.

Jerry often wondered what would have happened if his friends had not convinced him to get some help. During counseling, he had the chance to reflect on the concept of the vicious cycle. In his case, feelings of depression triggered heavy drinking. Heavy drinking made him physically sick, chronically tired and sleep-deprived, and even more depressed the next day. In that condition, he was unable to do his best at work or even to keep up his average level of performance. He was aware that his supervisor and even his coworkers were irritated with him. They had to carry more of the load and fix his mistakes, and this caused resentment. Having people angry at him increased his stress level and his depression. And he was then more likely to call his friends to go get drunk.

Getting help when he did began to reverse the vicious cycle into a kind of "healthy cycle." Once he began working on his mood, he didn't feel the need to drink as much as before. Once his drinking stayed at a healthy level, he no longer got sick from drinking, he could sleep better, and he was better rested during the day. His coworkers appreciated his being "all there" as he had been before. He felt needed and respected again. They could count on him again.

1. **If depressive moods are an issue for you, don't set as your goal *never* to experience negative moods again.** A more practical goal is to reduce their frequency, intensity, and duration—that is, how often they occur, how painful they are, and how long they last.

2. **Remember not to get depressed about being depressed.** Don't let depression demoralize you! This can happen if you begin to worry about why you aren't happier and to wonder if there is something wrong with you and if you will ever really get over this depression. Remember: negative mood is relatively common. It's unpleasant, but that's a reason to take it seriously, not to resent it.

3. **Remember that the task of learning to manage your moods is not yours alone.** Sometimes people with serious depression tell us they're tired of having to pay attention to their thoughts, their activities, and their contact with people. Why should they have to do this when other people do not? In fact, we believe that it's very useful to learn what affects your moods. Some people learn it more naturally, perhaps because they're exposed to people who do it well. Some actually notice that their moods are problematic early in life and begin to read about how to influence their own moods and to put what they read into practice. Some learn good ways to manage their moods, but, when something major happens, those ways are no longer enough, and they look for other ways to do so. So, if you feel burdened by the task of paying such close attention to your moods, try to remember that it's a task that everyone must undertake. It's just that you may have to learn to manage your own mood more systematically or later in life than others have. The task is still the same. We all have to learn to manage our moods.

> *Jenny suffered from depression, as did her mother and her grandmother. Having read about the genetics of depression, she assumed that she was genetically predisposed to being depressed. At first this knowledge had reduced her motivation to do anything about her depression. After all, it was in her genes. There was nothing she could do about that. However, one day she was talking to a friend who turned this idea on its head by sharing the following insight: People with genetic predispositions to depression actually are the ones who most need to learn how to manage their moods. People who are not predisposed to depression are less likely to suffer from negative moods, so they don't need the skills as much.*

The fact is that it's not clear how much of depression is influenced by our genes and how much is due to stressful events in our lives and the way we've learned to respond to them. Both are probably important. Either way, learning skills to keep your stress within a manageable range and your mood at a healthy level can't hurt.

Practical Ways to Manage Your Mood

If depression is causing you pain or life problems, a reasonable goal is to find practical ways to shorten the amount of time that you feel depressed. Psychologists interested in how depression occurs have found that people can learn to think in ways that help them prevent or get rid of depression. Here is a brief description of this approach. Other ways of managing your mood are described in Chapters 19, 20, 22, 24, 25, and 26.

Thinking Can Affect Depression

Often it's not what happens to you that makes you depressed, but rather how you choose to think about what happens. Here are two examples:

Martha invites Peter for dinner. Peter obviously does not like what she has cooked. Martha says to herself, "Oh, no, I never was a very good cook. What's the matter with me? I just can't do anything right!" Peter leaves early, she continues drinking until she falls asleep, and she is depressed about the whole thing for several days.

Mary invites John to dinner. John obviously does not like what she has cooked. Mary says to herself, "He must have pretty definite tastes." She decides to ask him what he likes next time. After dinner they have a pleasant evening together, sipping a special after-dinner wine. In the next few days, she has pleasant memories about the evening.

These two women had the same initial experience, but notice how differently they reacted to it. Martha took the situation personally and somehow inferred that Peter's distaste for the food reduced her worth. Mary, on the other hand, simply noted what had happened and considered how she might make it turn out better next time. Notice, too, that their reactions affected the rest of the evening, their drinking behavior, and even the days following the event.

How you think about things can affect how you end up feeling about them. To get a little practice in this, make a list of things that could happen to you and then think of at least two ways of looking at each of them—one that would make you feel good and one that would make you feel bad. Here are some examples:

Situation: "I just finished a tough job. It did not turn out well."
Negative interpretation: "I'm really a loser."
Positive interpretation: "It was a hard job, and I'll try another way next time."

Situation: "My conversation with Beth seemed boring."
Negative interpretation: "I guess I'm not very interesting to be with."
Positive interpretation: "I guess Beth and I don't have the same interests."

Situation: "I'm feeling down today."
Negative reaction: "Why does this always happen to me? I'm always depressed!"
Positive reaction: "I wonder what I can do to feel better?"

This is not a way of lying to yourself. If something unpleasant has happened, you need not hide from it, but neither do you need to consider it a terrible catastrophe. To manage your personal reality, you have to face reality. But there are many different ways to think about any situation, and you really can choose how to look at things from among many alternative points of view. Negative ways of seeing yourself and your life are not necessarily more accurate than positive ways of seeing yourself and your life. For example, in the first situation just presented, the fact that a job does not turn out well does not mean that you're a loser. Choosing to think so does, however, cause emotional pain. Even if you have faced a string of jobs that turned out badly, labeling yourself a loser is unlikely to do much good. "Facing reality" in this case could mean acknowledging that you need to change the way you do your work and coming up with a list of things you could do to improve your performance. Thinking this way will help you feel more optimistic and will increase the chances that you'll fare better next time. The more you learn to look for healthier ways of viewing things, the less time you'll have for the ways that make you feel bad without helping the situation. Even if you're responsible for an unpleasant event, you need not conclude that therefore you're a bad person.

Even if you're responsible for an unpleasant event, you need not conclude that therefore you're a bad person.

Summary

We have presented four important points that can be useful in coping with depression.

1. *Don't let depression itself demoralize you.* People who get depressed about being depressed promote a self-defeating spiral. Similarly, feeling resentful about having to learn to manage your mood ignores the fact that all of us have to continually learn this task.

2. *The way you think affects the way you feel.* There are several different ways of thinking about any situation, and you get to choose. Why not select a viewpoint that will make you feel better and will help you change in the future?

3. *Don't drink when you feel down.* Alcohol is a depressant drug, and although it may temporarily impair your brain enough to block out reality, it tends to make depression worse.

4. *Not all depression can be handled on your own.* If you find yourself experiencing many of the nine symptoms of major depression found in the Mood Screener (such as feeling down for a long time, eating less or much more, and having trouble sleeping because of depression), you should seek help from your primary-care physician or a psychologist or another mental health professional who specializes in the treatment of depression. Feeling down can also be related to physical illness. If there are indications that you may be ill, a medical checkup is a wise first step.

The Most Dangerous Symptom of Depression

One great danger from feelings of depression is the possibility that they might lead to suicidal ideas. The combination of depression and drinking can be particularly lethal. If you find yourself contemplating suicide,

People who seriously consider suicide often do not really want to die— they want their emotional pain to stop, and they can't think of an alternative.

you should definitely seek professional help. If you feel that you might hurt yourself at any moment, in the United States call 911 or the National Suicide Prevention Lifeline (1-800-273-8255), elsewhere try *www. befrienders.org* or go to the nearest emergency service for help. If you're beginning to consider suicide, call your local suicide prevention hotline. When one is seriously depressed, it is sometimes easy to convince oneself that suicide makes sense. Once the depression is over, people cannot imagine how they could have convinced themselves of that. Only those who make it through a suicidal period get the chance to see how mistaken they were, however, and how bright life can be on the other side of depression. Therefore, the focus during such times must be on obtaining help. Professionals who specialize in suicide prevention remark that people who seriously consider suicide do not really want to die—they want their emotional pain to stop, and they can't think of an alternative. But there are many alternatives now, and the pain can be addressed with professional help.

22

•

Self-Concept

Patricia had always been proud of her independent ways. She didn't let others tell her what to do. She didn't follow the crowd. She felt many of her school friends had sold out when they followed the usual paths to college or to start working for a big company. But, as time went on, she began to wonder whether she might have made a mistake. This came to a head once she began having children. Being unable to buy things for herself had never bothered her much. Her freedom was worth the inconvenience. But it was hard to tell her daughter Jeannie that she could not buy her a toy or take her to a movie. She was really devastated after her daughter entered school: Jeannie liked doing well in school, but when she needed help with homework, Patricia found the work difficult, particularly in math.

Patricia's image of herself as a free spirit and a rebel began to change into the image of an inadequate mother. At school events she began to feel inferior to the other parents, defensive about her lifestyle, and resentful about being pressured to conform for her daughter's sake. She began to drink prior to attending these events, and often after getting home from them, and after Jeannie went to sleep. But it was her deteriorating interactions with Jeannie when she had been drinking that finally convinced her to take action. She remembered something she had heard a long time ago: "If you don't change direction, you'll wind up where you are headed."

> If you don't change direction, you'll wind up where you are headed.

Self-concept refers to how you think about yourself, and *self-esteem* to how you feel about and value yourself. A negative self-concept and the feelings of worthlessness that accompany it sometimes lead to drinking. Alcohol provides a temporary escape from these unpleasant thoughts and feelings.

This chapter describes some alternatives: ways of building and maintaining a positive self-concept rather than running away from a negative one.

Your self-concept is an important part of your internal reality. It does not exist in the physical world. There is no way to observe it or measure it without asking you to describe it. Only you can change your self-concept or know when it has changed. Changing your self-concept involves shaping your internal reality, your mental world. Therefore, this chapter will focus on ways to mold the part of your internal reality most relevant to self-concept, namely, thoughts about yourself.

Feelings of worthlessness (low self-esteem) are usually enmeshed with negative thoughts about yourself (self-concept). If most thoughts about yourself are negative, then probably most feelings about yourself are also negative. One way of maintaining a positive self-concept is to increase your positive self-thoughts and decrease your negative self-thoughts. An image that can be helpful is to think of your internal environment as being similar in some ways to your external environment. Just as people are now attempting to reduce pollution and to rehabilitate areas of our world that have become toxic, so, too, can you identify those thoughts that are toxic to your self-concept and weed them out of your internal world, while planting and caring for those health-engendering thoughts that give you a sense of worth, a feeling of energy, a sense of being a good person. Of course, one way to increase positive thoughts about yourself is to store up positive things you have done so you can remember them in the future. So, a way to improve your internal (mental) world is to do things in your external (day-to-day) world that you can feel proud of.

Identify those thoughts that are toxic to your self-concept and weed them out of your internal world.

Increasing Positive Self-Thoughts

Set Up Reminders for Yourself

Thinking positive thoughts doesn't always come naturally. Sometimes it helps to have a reminder to think well of yourself. You could stick a piece of tape on the face of your watch, so that each time you check the time you will remember to think a positive thought. You might put a bit of colored tape on your cell phone or your key ring so that each time you use them you will be reminded. You can probably think of other possibilities that will fit your own lifestyle better.

The general idea is to use something that you do frequently to remind yourself to do something else that you are now doing less often. The effect of this method is even stronger if you practice doing the infrequent thing (in this case, think a positive thought about yourself) before you perform the more frequent behavior (for example, using your cell phone or keys).

Prime Yourself

Sometimes it's difficult to come up with positive self-thoughts spontaneously, especially if you're out of practice. For this reason it pays to sit down and make a list of positive remarks that apply to you. For example:

> "I'm a responsible person."
> "I'm a considerate person."
> "Many people like me."
> "I've been successful at keeping to my plan this week."
> "It has taken a lot of strength to deal with my problems."
> "I have good taste in clothes."
> "My family cares for me."
> "I love my kids."
> "I'm OK."

Make your own list of positive self-statements—at least 10 things you can say to yourself. Set up a reminder, and every time you see it, tell yourself something positive.

You can also try asking someone who knows and supports you to help you come up with a list of your positive characteristics. Perhaps you could say that you've been reading a book about how to improve your self-concept and the authors suggested you do this with a close friend. You could take turns coming up with positive characteristics you see in each other. On the facing page is a list of positive characteristics of people who succeed with change. Which of these are true of you? Why?

Go ahead—make your list!

My Positive Characteristics

1. _____

2. _____

3. _____

4. _____

5. _____

6. _____

7. _____

8. _____

9. _____

10. _____

Accepting	Committed	Flexible	Persevering	Stubborn
Active	Competent	Focused	Persistent	Thankful
Adaptable	Concerned	Forgiving	Positive	Thorough
Adventuresome	Confident	Forward-looking	Powerful	Thoughtful
Affectionate	Considerate	Free	Prayerful	Tough
Affirmative	Courageous	Happy	Quick	Trusting
Alert	Creative	Healthy	Reasonable	Trustworthy
Alive	Decisive	Hopeful	Receptive	Truthful
Ambitious	Dedicated	Imaginative	Relaxed	Understanding
Anchored	Determined	Ingenious	Reliable	Unique
Assertive	Die-hard	Intelligent	Resourceful	Unstoppable
Assured	Diligent	Knowledgeable	Responsible	Vigorous
Attentive	Doer	Loving	Sensible	Visionary
Bold	Eager	Mature	Skillful	Whole
Brave	Earnest	Open	Solid	Willing
Bright	Effective	Optimistic	Spiritual	Winning
Capable	Energetic	Orderly	Stable	Wise
Careful	Experienced	Organized	Steady	Worthy
Cheerful	Faithful	Patient	Straight	Zealous
Clever	Fearless	Perceptive	Strong	Zestful

Source: This list, compiled by Shelby Steen, is in the public domain. See Miller, W. R. (Ed.). (2004). *Combined behavioral intervention: A clinical research guide for therapists treating individuals with alcohol abuse and dependence* (COMBINE Monograph Series, Vol. 1). Bethesda, MD: National Institute on Alcohol Abuse and Alcoholism.

If there are positive characteristics you would like to have, but you don't think you can truthfully describe yourself as having them, consider gradually practicing those ways of acting. For example, if you would like to think of yourself as "considerate," begin acting thoughtfully toward others. Note when you do this so that next time you fill out this list you can honestly use that word to describe yourself.

Decreasing Negative Self-Thoughts

If, as your positive thoughts are increasing, you find that your negative self-thoughts are not decreasing, you can deal directly with them, too. One simple but surprisingly effective method is "thought stopping." When you become aware of a negative self-thought, imagine yourself yelling the word "Stop!" in your head as loudly as you can. It interrupts the negative thinking. Or tell yourself, "Thinking this way is hurtful to me. I choose instead to think differently." This, too, will interrupt the thought for a while. Better still, practice replacing toxic negative thoughts with positive self-statements.

> *Patricia really caught on to this method. She came into a counseling session one day with a big grin on her face and said she had come up with a way to remember what she was doing to herself and how to stop it: She had to stop using TNT on herself. She then explained that TNT stood for "Thinking Negative Thoughts."*

Negative self-thoughts are easy enough to recognize. Learn what your own negative thoughts are and become aware of when you start telling yourself such things as:

"Boy, am I dumb!"
"Everybody thinks I'm no good."
"I just don't have what it takes."
"I'm not very attractive."
"I could never be as good as _____."
"I'm too far gone to fix up my life."
"My life is ruined beyond repair."
"I'm too old to correct my mistakes."
"I'm hopeless."

"I'm a loser."

"I'm an alcoholic and I'll never change."

"Nobody could ever love me."

"I've hurt others so much, I don't deserve to be happy."

"What's the use?"

Notice that after even reading this list of negative thoughts you probably feel just a little more down or anxious. People often do. Imagine what having this type of thought numerous times throughout your day can do to your mood! Now try going back and reading through your list of 10 positive characteristics of yourself. Do you notice a change in how you feel?

As above, pay attention to whether you could change old patterns so that you no longer think of yourself as having these bad characteristics. For example, if you habitually hurt others, begin to be mindful when you are about to do so, and choose an alternative way to respond. After a while, it will no longer make sense to label yourself as someone who hurts others.

Setting Standards for Yourself

The standards that you set for yourself can also affect your self-concept. If you have established standards that are unrealistically high, you're inviting an unending series of disappointments. The more disappointed you become with yourself, the lower your self-esteem.

Unfortunately, there is no easy way to describe what are realistic standards. One possible guideline would be to set your standards high enough so that you need to exert a healthy effort to achieve them, but not so high that they are constantly beyond your reach.

Setting standards, by the way, is not limited to work situations. You set standards for yourself in many areas, sometimes without being aware of doing so. These areas may include your home, work, education, social life, spiritual life, sex life, physical condition, and leisure activities.

If your high standards come in the form of long-range goals, it may help to break them down into smaller steps. Gradual change that takes moderate, sustained effort is often easier to maintain than dramatic change that takes "all you've got" or more. It is hard to maintain an all-out effort for very long. If, for example, you have a standard (goal) for yourself to be 50 pounds lighter and tell yourself you cannot be happy until you've reached that goal, you'll be unhappy for a long time. If you adjust your standards so that every step in the right direction makes you happy, you're likely to feel better sooner. You're also more likely to reach your eventual goal. For example, if you set a goal of reducing your weight at the rate of 1 pound per week, you will be more likely to succeed. In a year, you will have reached your overall objective, and you will be more likely to keep your weight steady.

Gradual change that takes moderate, sustained effort is often easier to maintain than dramatic change that takes "all you've got."

Patricia wished she had done some things differently, but overall she felt comfortable with having lived up to her own values. Her daughter might grow up to have a different point of view from hers, and Patricia would have to learn to understand and respect it. After all, it had really bothered her when her own mother tried to convince her to think as she did. She did not want to do that to Jeannie. On the other hand, there were things she could teach Jeannie that would probably come in handy in life, but to do that she would have to feel more comfortable with herself. She decided to begin this process by molding the thoughts she had when she was with other parents so she could feel more at ease in their company. After all, if Jeannie saw her being defensive, she would begin thinking her mother had reason to be defensive. If she saw her being confident and comfortable with herself, she would continue to see her mother as a competent adult, as she had when she was a small child. Patricia still remembered the time they had solved a problem together and Jeannie had looked at her with those big eyes of hers full of wonder and admiration and said with all the certainty of a 4-year-old: "Mommy, you are so smart!"

Although we cannot give you clear guidelines for deciding on realistic standards for yourself, we can point to danger signs that may mean you've set your sights too high. If you notice that you're constantly failing to reach goals you set for yourself and that unpleasant feelings result, reexamine your personal standards. Negative emotional reactions are natural when you're disappointed. They become dangerous when they happen again and again and begin to produce effects such as depression, sleep loss, marked weight loss or weight gain, relationship difficulties, violent behavior, physical symptoms, or overdrinking.

A pole vaulter charges down the practice track, launches into the air, and fails to clear the bar, bringing it down into the sawdust. There are two ways of looking at it: The vaulter wasn't good enough. Or the bar was a little too high.

On Perfectionism

A common source of low self-concept is perfectionism. More specifically, it's the belief that if you're not perfect, you're a failure. This belief can have substantial impact on both internal and external reality. It can be a source of significant emotional pain, and it can also keep you from realizing your potential. Fear of not doing things perfectly can result in not doing them at all. The well-known saying "Don't let the perfect be the enemy of the good" suggests that perfectionism can get in the way of doing some very good things. Edmund Burke said it well: "Nobody made a greater mistake than he who did nothing because he could only do a little."

> *Don't let the perfect be the enemy of the good.*

This does not mean that you shouldn't try to be your best or to improve on what you've done before. Perfection is unattainable, but it can be a useful guiding star. In past centuries those who sailed the seas using guiding stars never expected to reach those stars. The stars gave them a direction, not a destination.

One final word from the ancient Greeks may be helpful here. The Greek word *telos* is sometimes translated as "perfect," but it actually refers to the natural, mature end state. An oak tree is the telos of a particular acorn. No two oak trees are exactly alike, but each can be perfect in this sense—the natural, fully developed tree that was waiting in the acorn.

Patricia continued using the priming technique to remind herself of the many positive characteristics she had built up over the years. The characteristics identified from the list earlier in the chapter were that she was adventuresome, affectionate, alive, assertive, brave, clever, courageous, die-hard, fearless, free, happy, powerful, resourceful, stubborn, tough, unstoppable, and zestful. That was the kind of person she had wanted to be since she was very young, and she had become what she wanted. She consciously reminded herself that if she were able to help Jeannie develop even half of these characteristics, Jeannie would be a formidable person. If, in addition, Jeannie wanted to follow the more traveled route, that was OK with Patricia. After all, freedom was a very high value for her, and Jeannie should be free to construct her own life.

Patricia also began to do things that would make it possible to label herself (honestly) as ambitious, capable, persevering, and relaxed. She had begun using some online tools to learn more math, so she could help Jeannie with her homework. It was hard at first, but as she kept at it she began to grasp the material and felt proud of herself as she did so. She also began to focus on the other parents at school functions, asking them about their interests, instead of just feeling defensive about her own. This helped her relax and actually enjoy these interactions.

As the weeks passed, and thinking this way became second nature to her, Patricia noticed that the other parents tended to seek her out. She was, after all, different from them. And now that her happiness and vitality were more evident, she began to notice a certain wistfulness in some of the other mothers, almost as though they envied her having followed another path. She thought she saw Jeannie giving her looks of pride from time to time—or perhaps she imagined it. Either way, her relationship with Jeannie had improved a lot. Patricia's drinking had gone back to her usual moderate level, and there hadn't been any more drinking-related conflicts.

23

•

Sleeping Well

It was 1:00 in the morning, and Wendy lay awake in the darkness of her bedroom. For 2 hours she had been trying to get to sleep, but thoughts kept racing through her mind, and although she felt weary she just couldn't seem to let go. Often when this happened to her she had tried turning on the light and reading detective stories for a while, but usually that hadn't worked. Counting sheep only bored her until she began thinking about something else again. But there was one thing that almost always worked. . . .

One hour and 6 ounces (177 ml) of gin later, Wendy was fast asleep. Somehow the alcohol seemed to help her relax and unwind, to let go of the day and shut off her racing thoughts. Even so, she would toss and turn through the night, and when she awakened the next morning, she felt unrested and vaguely irritable. Her weariness would catch up with her in midafternoon, when she would nap for an hour or two. Then came the next evening, and it started all over again. Wendy had begun to dread the nighttime, the long hours of trying to get to sleep, and the half-remembered disturbing dreams that sometimes followed.

Sleeping well is often called "sleeping like a baby." Unfortunately, what was once a natural ability seems to elude many adults. The term *insomnia* refers to a set of common problems in getting to sleep or staying asleep. About one person in four is troubled by frequent insomnia. Among people seeking help with alcohol, the percentage seems to be even higher.

Insomnia has many different causes. Sometimes it results from a specific medical problem. It can be related to depression or to stress. When alcohol is involved, the picture becomes even more complicated. Some people believe they need to drink to fall

One in four adults suffers from frequent insomnia.

asleep, yet it's entirely possible that drinking is contributing to the sleep disturbance—a vicious cycle that can make you miserable.

Think about it: Given that there are 24 hours in a day, if you sleep 6 hours a night, you are spending a quarter of your life sleeping. If you sleep 8 hours a night, you are spending a third of your life sleeping. If the experience of sleep is frustrating, if your sleep is not restful, if you toss and turn because you cannot sleep, then a good chunk of your life and personal reality is unpleasant at best. If drinking has caused or contributed to problems with sleeping for you, learning to sleep without using alcohol is key. Managing this part of your daily reality can improve your physical and mental health. And eliminating the need for alcohol to sleep is another good step in managing your drinking.

Alcohol and Sleep

Many people find that alcohol seems to help them get to sleep. Indeed, anything that induces relaxation seems to be helpful in falling asleep. The problem is that alcohol's effects do not end there.

Alcohol is a drug that interferes with the normal sleep cycle in complicated ways. If you're sleeping with alcohol in your bloodstream, you may not get enough of the deepest, most restful kind of sleep and thus may wake in the morning feeling unrested. Alcohol also seems to interfere with dreaming, an important part of normal sleep. Alcohol in the bloodstream at least partially suppresses dreaming. As the blood alcohol level decreases, however, there may be a kind of "rebound" of dreaming. Many of our clients have reported intense periods of dreaming or nightmares during early morning, when blood alcohol levels are dropping. Finally, alcohol seems to make it more likely that a person will be restless during sleep and will wake up more frequently during the night. Not everyone who drinks experiences all of these effects, but in general this holds: although alcohol may help you fall asleep, it tends to cause your sleep to be disturbed and abnormal.

Thus alcohol and other sedating drugs are not good treatments for most kinds of insomnia in the long run. Furthermore, a pattern of drinking to get to sleep can gradually escalate, causing threats to health or other life problems. If you have been using alcohol to help you sleep, we strongly recommend that you seek another way to sleep well.

It is also worth mentioning here that when a person has become accustomed or addicted to alcohol and then decreases or stops drinking, insomnia frequently occurs as part of the withdrawal from alcohol. If you don't understand what is happening, you may be tempted to use alcohol again to get to sleep, but that only prolongs the problem. In our experience this kind of acute insomnia, which begins when a person decreases drinking, often passes within a few weeks and is not reason for great concern (except, of course, that it indicates some physical dependence on alcohol).

Coping with Insomnia

A number of strategies seem to be helpful to people suffering from the common varieties of insomnia. We focus primarily on methods to help you fall asleep more quickly, although we briefly discuss nighttime awakening and nightmares as well.

Relaxation

Falling asleep is perfectly natural, not something that you have to will or learn how to do. When you're tired, you naturally fall asleep unless there are obstacles that block this process. Coping with normal insomnia, then, is more a matter of removing obstacles than of learning how to "make yourself" fall asleep.

The relaxation skills described in Chapter 18 can help. Relaxing helps to remove the tensions of the day. Indeed, research indicates that practicing relaxation at bedtime can be helpful to people suffering from insomnia. If you're a newcomer to the methods in Chapter 18, try going through the tension–relaxation exercises for all the muscle groups before falling asleep. Once you're relaxed physically, you may fall asleep naturally. The goal here is to focus on relaxing your body and your mind, *not* to "make yourself" go to sleep. After completing the exercises, just continue to enjoy the feelings of deep relaxation, feelings that are compatible with sleeping.

Incidentally, practicing relaxation *only* at bedtime may inadvertently teach you to feel sleepy whenever you relax, which you might not find desirable. So start doing the relaxation exercises at other times during the day as well, when you're not getting ready to go to sleep.

Developing a Regular Daily Rhythm

Your body works best when you operate on a predictable cycle of activity and rest. If you continually change the times of day when you sleep, your body cannot settle into a regular cycle. Another way to improve your sleep, then, is to pick a regular bedtime and waking time and stick to these as much as possible so you synchronize your biological clock. Turn in at about the same time every night and set your alarm for about the same time every morning. This does not rule out the occasional late nights or mornings of sleeping in, but the more regular you can make your sleep time, the better.

The best way to improve your sleep is to pick a regular bedtime and waking time and stick to these as much as possible so you synchronize your biological clock.

It may also be helpful to schedule your daily activities so that you begin to slow down as bedtime nears. Parents recognize the importance of this tactic with their children: no arousing or stimulating play just before bedtime. This can be an important factor in your own sleep. Try not to spend the hour before bedtime in activities that require intensive planning, that stimulate many thoughts or worries. This is time for winding down. If you drink coffee or other beverages with caffeine, experiment with eliminating these stimulants in the evening.

What's a Bed for, Anyway?

A third strategy that has been found to be helpful is to avoid using your bed for anything except sleeping. Often people who have trouble getting to sleep will turn on the light and read in bed or will lie and think in bed and plan the next day. Some people eat in bed or watch television through their toes. If you're in this habit, get out of bed and go to another room if possible whenever you want to read or eat or think or plan. You should associate bed with falling asleep. (An obvious exception to this is sex, but that's just fine. Bed is for sleeping and for sex and nothing else.) Of course some people are perfectly able to read or watch television in bed and then quickly fall asleep, and for them it's no problem. If you suffer from insomnia, however, this strategy can be very helpful. Try it!

Don't Lie There Awake

This strategy is related to the last one: It is not helpful to lie awake in bed "trying" to get to sleep. If you are not falling asleep and you are becoming emotionally upset about it, get up, leave the bedroom, and do something else.

One way to use this strategy is to choose a length of time that seems reasonable for you to get to sleep. Probably this should not be shorter than

10 minutes or longer than 30 minutes. If, after you retire for the night, you have not fallen asleep during this amount of time, get up and out of bed. Go do something else until you feel sleepy. When you start to feel sleepy, go back to bed, practice relaxation, and allow yourself to fall asleep. If again you are not asleep within the "reasonable" time you have chosen, get up again and start over. Some people find it helpful to get completely dressed when they get up, marking the difference between being awake and falling asleep.

There are two other rules to observe if this strategy is to work for you. First of all, set your alarm and get up at the same time each morning, no matter how many times you've been up during the night or how tired you feel. Second, do not allow yourself to nap during the day. Remember that the goal is to establish a regular sleep cycle. Sleeping late or napping will defeat this purpose.

During the first few days of using this strategy, you may find that you are getting up a number of times. This can be frustrating, but so is lying there awake. Usually within a week or so your body's need for a regular sleep cycle will take over, and the strategy will begin to pay off.

Getting It All Together

These four strategies work best when they are used together, although they are of some help individually as well. If you want to work on sleeping better, we recommend that you start all of these strategies on a selected night (How about tonight?). Choose regular times to go to bed and to awaken in the morning and honor these. Choose a reasonable amount of time to fall asleep. Practice relaxation when you turn in, remembering that your goal is to become deeply relaxed. Don't "work" on going to sleep. It's more a process of letting go, of allowing sleep to happen. If you are not getting to sleep, get up and do something else for a while. Don't lie awake and don't read, eat, watch television, or play games while lying in bed. Get out of bed, do something else, and return when sleepy. Regardless of these times out of bed, get up at the prescribed time in the morning, and no napping during the day!

Nighttime Awakening

Another problem that people can have with sleep is awakening in the middle of the night and not being able to get back to sleep. A few bits of knowledge may help here.

First of all, you should know that it is perfectly normal to wake up briefly during the night. The body cycles through several stages of deep and light sleep, and sometimes in light sleep one awakens briefly. This seems to happen more often as people age.

Second, the fact that you've awakened does not mean you'll stay awake. Sometimes when people find themselves awake in the night they start saying things to themselves like "Oh no! Now I'm awake and I won't be able to go back to sleep again! Why does this always have to happen to me?" Such thoughts are upsetting and tend to cause you to wake up further. It's much better to tell yourself something like "Oh, I'm awake. That's natural, and soon I'll be asleep again. Just relax."

Your relaxation skills can also be used at these times, just as you use them in falling asleep initially. Rather than thinking about waking up or focusing your thoughts on something that will arouse you, just relax yourself and let your body help you drift back to sleep. Let go of whatever thoughts enter your mind: there's no need to pursue them or to keep on thinking about them. Just let your thoughts go and continue to relax.

> *Arnold, who suffered from alcohol-related sleep problems, eventually told us that one of the helpful thoughts he came up with was "I can enjoy being relaxed in bed, even if I'm not sleeping." Thinking this helped him reduce the feelings of frustration he had generally felt before when he was tossing and turning in bed, looking at the numerals on the bedside clock. He also mentioned that this was easier to do when the bedroom was comfortably cool.*

People who suffer from insomnia and who have successfully solved this problem recount many other strategies:

- Don't drink fluids just before going to bed so you won't have to wake up to go to the bathroom.
- Definitely don't drink anything containing caffeine after 2:00 P.M.
- Don't drink alcohol within 2 hours of your bedtime.
- Don't smoke or use other drugs within 2 hours of your bedtime.
- Don't exercise within 3 hours of your bedtime.
- If you wake up in the middle of the night, don't have a snack; your body may learn to feel hungry in the middle of the night, and hunger can wake you up.
- Make your sleep environment comfortable: reduce noise (use earplugs if necessary) or use something that generates gentle white noise, darken the room (use a sleeping mask if necessary), and arrange for a comfortable room temperature.

- If it happens that you wake up and are lying awake for more than the reasonable time you have chosen, get out of bed and return to it only when you feel sleepy.

Nightmares

Some people suffer from insomnia because they have regular nightmares that awaken them and leave them feeling upset. It can be hard to go back to sleep when you're jolted awake with a pounding heart, rapid breathing, and feeling cold or sweating (or both). People who have this experience night after night can naturally end up wary of falling asleep to begin with and may use alcohol to lull them into sleep.

Good science is accumulating on nightmares. They can be related to tension level. People going to sleep in a state of muscle tension may be more likely to have a nightmare. For this reason people often learn that a drug that induces relaxation (as alcohol does in moderate doses) may make nightmares less likely to occur. Relaxation training can help significantly. One of the treatment strategies that we tried was teaching people the relaxation skills described in Chapter 18. This proved to be just as helpful as a more extensive treatment method.[23] A number of people suffering from frequent and severe nightmares showed substantial or complete improvement after learning relaxation.

By the way, some people who have nightmares are also concerned that the nightmares mean there is something wrong with their mental health. This is rarely the case. Many of the people treated in our nightmare research program had suffered from severe nightmares for many years but showed no abnormal personality patterns or other major psychological problems.

Do You Need Additional Help?

Some sleep problems require more extensive treatment and professional attention. If you've tried relaxation for a few weeks, along with the other strategies mentioned in this chapter, without improvement in your insomnia, you may want to seek additional help. Many cities now have a hospital or university with a sleep clinic at which specialists treat these common problems. Your local medical center, a university psychology department, or your personal physician may be able to help you locate a qualified specialist.

24

•

Mindfulness

Dante started drinking in high school. He found that it helped him deal with feeling overwhelmed by life and then feeling depressed by the conclusion that he didn't have what it takes to be successful. He assumed that unless he met his major goals, he was worthless, and these thoughts often reverberated in his head. Psychologists call this "ruminating"—going over and over the same painful ideas so that they drain one's energy and sometimes lead to repeated episodes of serious depression.

As Dante entered adulthood, depression and drinking seemed to go hand in hand. The more he drank, the more depressed he became. The more depressed he felt, the more he drank. Eventually he was treated for depression several times, and he responded well to antidepressants. Yet as time went on, the periods of normal mood between depressions seemed to get shorter and shorter. During his most recent episode of depression his psychiatrist suggested he try a new "maintenance" treatment, one that had been found useful in preventing recurrences of depression. This new treatment was called "mindfulness-based cognitive therapy." Once he found out that the treatment involved learning to meditate and having to commit to an ongoing meditation practice, he was very reluctant to try it. After all, he said, he had already learned and tried all the relaxation methods that were supposed to distract him from the self-blame that wound him up and led to drinking and more depression. His doctor explained that, although mindfulness meditation could result in a state of relaxation, that was not its primary goal. Instead, it was intended to help people become more aware, and perhaps even accepting, of their experience in the moment so that they might choose to react differently, rather than continuing to be at the mercy of their habitual knee-jerk behaviors—which in Dante's case involved overdrinking.

Dante remained skeptical, but because medication seemed to work only when he was actively depressed, without preventing another episode, he decided almost anything was worth a try. He was tired of having his life overtaken by his mood. To his surprise, Dante found that he was able to use the meditation skills he learned to become less overwhelmed by his own thoughts. One of the things he learned was to just observe his thoughts as they appeared, without judging them, and to do so while generating feelings of kindness and compassion toward himself. The more he practiced these skills, the less the thoughts prompted feelings of depression, and the less he felt a need to drink. He learned to observe his urges to drink without judging them, and without having to act on them. Each urge was just another event in his mind, which was interesting, but which did not have to move him to feel bad or to do something he had chosen not to do. Just as he was learning to observe his thoughts and his cravings without judging them, he began to observe himself without judging himself. As his feelings of depression became less intense and less frequent, he was able to become more mindful about his drinking, so that it no longer occurred automatically.

The Benefits of Living Mindfully

The approach to moderation laid out in this book is based in the value of mindful living. Twenty-five hundred years after Socrates said "The unexamined life is not worth living," Viktor Frankl pointed out that the examined life comes with the power to make choices: "Between stimulus and response there is a space. In that space is our power to choose our response. In our response lies our growth and our freedom." As Dante discovered, getting out of automatic pilot can mean freeing oneself from habits like overdrinking.

Dante benefited from a fortuitous melding of Western and Eastern thought that has occurred in the last few decades. Ancient meditation practices from Asia demonstrated one effective way to achieve mindfulness, and treatments integrating these practices with Western science, such as mindfulness-based stress reduction (MBSR), mindfulness-based cognitive therapy (MBCT), and finally mindfulness-based relapse prevention for addictive behaviors (MBRP), have helped many people cope with medical illnesses, pain, mood disorders, and substance use. MBCT has been proven effective in reducing recurrences of depression, especially in individuals like Dante who have had several episodes. MBCT uses methods from cognitive-behavioral therapy to help people challenge their unhelpful thoughts, along with meditation to help them achieve *aware-ness* and *equanimity*. MBRP also joins cognitive-behavioral therapy with relapse prevention strategies to help people in recovery increase their awareness of trig-gers and habitual reactions, to create a new relationship with these experiences, and to develop specific skills to use when faced with

> *Mindful living is learning to achieve awareness and equanimity.*

high-risk situations. These approaches are also invaluable to people who are moderating their drinking and face situations that might entice them to drink more than they want or to engage in risky behaviors in general.

Awareness

Most people believe they are generally aware of their environment and their own responses to it. If they weren't, how would they manage to cross the street safely, complete errands and chores, and get to work on time? The fact is, many routine tasks are conducted on autopilot. How often have you found yourself on the other side of the street or back home from going on an errand without any memory of walking or driving? The ability to multitask may seem like a boon to efficiency—What's wrong with plan-ning your presentation for the next sales meeting while you mindlessly fold the laundry?—but it comes at a cost. Recent research has in fact shown that the ability to multitask may be more myth than reality—that we can't really do two things at once without one of them suffering. Things get even worse when we reflexively react to certain emotions and thoughts with behavior that disserves us. Overdrinking is a prime example. In Dante's case, whenever he started to ruminate about his "worthlessness," feelings of depression would overtake him and, without consciously thinking about it, he would reach for a beer.

In terms of moderate drinking, awareness might involve being con-sciously aware:

- That you are being offered a drink,
- Whether you are feeling like accepting the drink or not,
- Whether doing so is in accord with the choice you have made as part of your drinking plan, and
- That you can consciously choose to accept the drink or not.

Increasing awareness of each of these moments would increase the likeli-hood that you will reach your goals. In specific cases like Dante's, increasing awareness of the downward spiral of rumination that traps him might give him the space between stimulus and response that would lead to a choice *not* to reach for a beer.

Equanimity

Equanimity refers to a state of emotional stability, of not being "moved" by automatic emotional responses to events (either positive or negative), of being able to set aside the tendency to judge yourself or others. Equanimity enhances awareness in the sense that, after you perceive whatever is going on within your mind and body, as well as in the outside world, you are not distracted by your attachment to specific goals or aversion to specific things or events. You can be a witness to what is going on without judging it, and thus be less likely to react automatically. Your sense of freedom to live your life the way you have chosen yourself becomes stronger. You feel less buffeted by your usual knee-jerk reactions and more able to truly make a conscious choice. Practicing mindfulness meditation allowed Dante to recognize his pattern of blaming himself for "not measuring up," self-criticism that was so painful to him that he automatically tried to drown it in alcohol.

Mindfulness meditation can be thought of as inserting a step between the stimulus of a destructive emotion and the response of drinking alcohol.

Equanimity is increased through meditation because in meditating you learn to observe every part of your experience without judging it. As you observe thoughts moving past the window of your mind like floating clouds, for example, you gradually realize that a thought is just a thought. A thought is not reality. Thoughts are created by your own mind, based on what you have learned throughout your life. You do not have to react to every thought you have, including (and especially) the thoughts that can cause you the most distress and the most pain. Similarly, emotions do not require automatic, active responses. They can be observed in the same way thoughts are. You eventually learn that the fact that you are anxious or terrified does not necessarily mean that anything terrible is going to happen to you. Sometimes it just means that you are anxious or terrified. Just becoming aware of that can sometimes help reduce your fear.

Acceptance is a key element that is implied in mindfulness meditation. Several therapists have pointed out that when efforts to change your negative patterns of thinking or behavior do not yield success, and when you become desperate, your frenzied efforts can exacerbate the problem. You may begin to avoid situations that are difficult or give up on your efforts to change. The focus on nonjudgmental awareness of the reality inside you and around you helps reduce the potential demoralization that a rigid focus on change can sometimes produce. Acceptance refers to being able to see things as they are, with equanimity, rather than with your usual emotional or behavioral reaction (such as getting angry or depressed and looking for a drink). To change a reality that would be good for you to change, you must first face the reality just as it is, without sugar-coating it, or making excuses, and without overreacting to it. Only then can you mindfully choose what you will do given the actual circumstances (rather than merely wishing that things were different or being resentful about the way things are).

Practicing Mindfulness Meditation

Studies show that mindfulness meditation produces many changes in brain wave activity, cerebral blood flow, and release of neurotransmitters. These changes have been interpreted as increasing an individual's ability to be alert, focus attention, relax, and reduce compulsive behavior. These abilities can go a long way toward helping you reach your goal of moderate drinking. You can learn to witness the passing of thoughts and desires that ordinarily lead you to drink by suspending judgment of those thoughts and feelings and of yourself. You can learn to accept life as it is, without striving to change it and without becoming frantic when you do not reach your goals—including the goal of moderating your drinking. Being able to renew your efforts without getting down on yourself for repetitions of overdrinking can facilitate lasting change.

Obviously, old habits are hard to break, and the benefits of mindfulness meditation do not accrue to anyone overnight. Mindfulness takes practice. Many experts believe the best results come from regular formal meditation practice, preferably following training by a qualified teacher. It is possible, however, to learn mindfulness meditation on your own, and to practice it in an informal way throughout the day rather than at scheduled times. The Resources at the back of this book can steer you to several good self-help books on the subject, as well as to some websites with additional information and support. Meanwhile, though, there are a few things you can try to give yourself a taste of a new awareness and equanimity that might change the role you assign to alcohol in your life.

Mindful Breathing

If there is one experience we pay little attention to it's the action of breathing. Many mindfulness meditation programs start with helping participants breathe in a mindful way. To get a sense of what this feels like, try this simplified version for a minute right now:

Sit or lie down in a quiet setting, with your eyes closed or focused a few feet in front of you. Allow your breath to flow naturally, in and out, as you turn your attention to the experience of inhaling and exhaling. You can focus not only on the action of breathing, but also on the sensory experience: the temperature of the air as it enters or leaves your nostrils, the change in pressure in your chest, the moment at which your lungs turn from inhaling to exhaling. Meditation teachers explain to novices that their mind will drift. There is nothing wrong with that. In fact, that's the whole point. You become mindfully aware that you have drifted, and then you bring yourself back to a focus on your breath without criticizing yourself for having drifted. If you can, do this for about 20 minutes. You will be surprised by what you notice about this simple, automatic act. You will probably also be surprised by the thoughts that float through your mind, distracting your attention from your breath to a number of other concerns. This little exercise can be a revelation about how fickle our attention can be and how incomplete our awareness.

Practicing the breathing exercise can be extremely valuable to your efforts to avoid being carried away by the impulse to overdrink. Many experts advocate use of what is called the "3-minute breathing space," in which you respond to a feeling of anxiety or an urge to drink by taking 3 minutes to breathe mindfully—creating a space between stimulus and response in action.

The Body Scan

A common next step in mindfulness meditation practice is an exercise known as the "body scan." The purpose of this practice is to help people reclaim their ability to be aware of all of their bodily experience. We have all learned to ignore minor aches and pains on the one hand and to quickly scratch every itch on the other. What is lost in the process is the ability to be fully aware of the full richness of one's experience in any given moment. Without that expansive awareness, it's difficult to make fully informed choices.

THE SOBER BREATHING SPACE

One way to bring mindfulness into your life that can help you cope with daily challenges is an exercise you can do anywhere and at any time. It is called the SOBER breathing space, and it can be used if you are moderating your drinking or have decided to quit entirely.

- <u>S</u>top or slow down right where you are and bring awareness to this moment.

- <u>O</u>bserve what is happening in this moment, in your body, your emotions, and your thoughts.

- <u>B</u>reathe and notice the sensations of the in-breath and the out-breath.

- <u>E</u>xpand awareness to the reactions in your body to the situation you are in.

- <u>R</u>espond mindfully and choose a course of action. Do not judge your choice.

This exercise is somewhat similar to progressive relaxation (Chapter 18), but instead of tensing and releasing the muscles in each body part, you simply focus your attention on one body part at a time and, with gentle interest and curiosity, notice all the sensations that come from it. To get a taste of this practice, try a little of it right now. It's customary to start with the breathing exercise above. Then focus on one body part, typically either a part of one foot or a part of your head, and observe all the shifting sensations there before moving either up or down your body to each successive part. You can also continue to focus on sounds, smells, and eventually your own thoughts and emotions. Merely become aware of all these sensations, without trying to change them, and without judging them. You might consider each thought or sensation as a bird flying past the open window of your mind or a cloud floating by in the sky. Unpleasant sensations should not be avoided, but merely observed. Some professionals believe this practice might reduce the impact of such sensations, making it easier to bear them at other times. If you're trying to moderate your drinking, the acute awareness and acceptance you might develop through the body scan could allow you to tolerate anxiety, shame, pain, or any other discomfort that you have been trying to manage by anesthetizing it with alcohol.

Eating Meditations

Another way to practice mindfulness is to start eating mindfully. A time-honored example called the "raisin exercise" is a good way to get started. Again, more complete instructions are available in numerous sources such as those listed in the Resources, but what the practice amounts to is this, which you can try for yourself: Take a single raisin and instead of popping it into your mouth, taking a couple of chews and swallowing without much thought, really experience the raisin with all your senses. You might start by picking up the raisin and noticing how it feels and looks. Take your time and really look at it and touch it. Then put it in your mouth and just observe how it feels in your mouth. Now feel it all over with your tongue. Again, take your time and notice the texture, scent, and taste before you slowly chew and then swallow it. Many people who try this simple exercise discover to their astonishment that this little shriveled dried fruit is nothing like what they had thought of as a raisin before.

URGE SURFING

Another technique using visualization and mindfulness has proved very helpful in high-risk situations. Urge surfing is a method practiced in advance of a situation in which you know you might be triggered to overdrink. The first step is to picture yourself in a situation in your present life, say when your ex-husband is going to be attending the same cocktail party and you know he is likely to bring his new girlfriend. Close your eyes, or leave them slightly open, staring at a place on the floor, and then imagine yourself at the party. Breathing easily, bring yourself to that exact moment in which you will feel triggered to have that extra drink, perhaps when you see your ex and his partner. What emotions are arising? What thoughts are going through your mind? Do you feel weak at the knees or lightheaded? If you can, notice what feels intolerable about the situation and try to stay with those difficult feelings, riding the crest of the wave, and down the other side, until the feelings subside. Just the practice of riding the wave until the feelings subside can increase your confidence that you'll respond mindfully in a challenging moment in your daily life. By practicing how to tolerate the difficult feelings, you can more easily resist triggers. This may not work every time, but it is yet another useful tool to have in your box when you know you're entering a challenging situation.

This is one area where you can easily focus an informal mindfulness practice. Instead of bolting a fast-food meal between tasks, try sitting down to a meal at least once a day and really paying attention to the experience of eating. Many people find that their appreciation for the food is so greatly enhanced that they actually eat less. You can choose to mindfully drink a glass of wine, for example, taking a sip, feeling it slip down your throat, placing the glass back down on the table, and enjoying the sensation of drinking a glass slowly.

We hope the information we have given you here provides enough glimpses into the mindfulness approach to health to inoculate you from some of the down sides of being excessively focused on major changes, and make you curious enough to explore mindfulness approaches that could be helpful in your life. Mindfulness meditation is one approach that can be taken step by step and provide you with many tools with which to challenge habitual choices, notice triggers, observe your response, and choose instead to respond mindfully.

25

Managing Anxiety and Fear

Michelle's job requires her to make public presentations from time to time. This was not part of the job description when she was hired, but a few promotions later it has become part of her routine. She never would have taken the position if she had known that talking in front of large audiences would be required. She has a strong fear of public speaking. Now she finds herself increasingly anxious as the day of a presentation approaches. Lately she has found herself carrying a bottle of vodka in her car and taking a couple of swigs before she walks into the auditorium. She's starting to feel completely dependent on this liquid courage to fulfill an important job responsibility, but what if someone sees her drinking in her car? Michelle is worried that she'll get labeled as a secret alcoholic and end up fired. But if she can't make her presentations, she'll surely lose her job. What can she do?

As discussed in Chapter 18, alcohol is sometimes used to relieve tension. There are also discomforts much more intense than simple tension, described by such words as *anxiety, fear, panic, distress,* and *dread.* Everyone needs a way to cope with such strong feelings. Alcohol is sometimes used for this purpose.

For example:

Do you feel you need a drink to be comfortable in social situations?
Do you fortify yourself with a drink before making a difficult phone call or before broaching a topic that you fear will incur someone's wrath?
Does it take a few beers to be able to speak your mind?
Do you need some alcohol before you can engage in romantic or sexual activities, to get beyond fears or hesitations?
Do you drink to escape from painful memories?

Do you have to build courage with a drink to face heavy responsibilities?

Do you feel severe discomfort in certain situations?

Do you worry a lot, sometimes long before the feared event?

Do you obsess about

- having to talk in front of a large number of people?
- the possibility of being fired?
- the possible end of a close personal relationship?

Do you find yourself in severe discomfort during adjustment periods? For example,

- going through a divorce?
- working against deadlines?
- looking for a job?

Have you developed specific fears, such as a fear of

- negative evaluation or rejection?
- flying in airplanes?
- being alone?

Do you find yourself experiencing severe discomfort after a critical or traumatic event has passed, in the form of residual tension or painful memories?

Do your memories of the event come in the form of feelings of failure, frustration, loss, or even outright panic?

If these feelings are so intense that they are interfering with your life or activities a lot, consult a professional behavior therapist trained to deal with these highly treatable problems of anxiety, panic, or posttraumatic stress. Using alcohol to cope with them is clearly insufficient and often produces additional problems. If, on the other hand, the anxious feelings are merely uncomfortable but still trigger undesired drinking, the ideas in this chapter may be helpful.

One way to get through difficult situations is to increase your ability to deal with them. By increasing your competence you also increase your sense of power over your own life and raise your self-confidence. Learning skills to handle life situations makes those situations less fearful. Some skills that are useful for handling various life situations are discussed in later chapters, such as the ability to be assertive and the ability to relate to others.

Another way to cope with stressful situations is to make them less frightening so that you can

Learning skills to handle life situations makes those situations less fearful.

handle them more easily. Making yourself less fearful really means making yourself less sensitive to a particular kind of situation—that is, *desensitizing* yourself to it. The process of desensitization can be accomplished through a relatively straightforward method, if followed systematically.

Systematic Desensitization

Systematic desensitization makes use of the relaxation skills described in Chapter 18. Remember that anxiety and fear involve both mental and muscular tension. Your muscles tighten when you anticipate some kind of pain. By physically relaxing your muscles, you can short-circuit anxiety. Relaxation and anxiety are physiologically incompatible; it's difficult to experience both at the same time.

To explain desensitization requires adding another idea to the relaxation method. This is the concept of a *gradual approach*. If you are repeatedly faced with a mildly threatening situation, you eventually get used to it and no longer feel anxious. You can then proceed to a slightly more threatening situation, until you become immune to it, and so on, until a formerly overwhelming situation becomes manageable. Systematic desensitization involves using your relaxation skills in combination with the gradual approach. You present yourself with the difficult situation while you are calm and deeply relaxed, and present it in such a way that you approach it gradually. In this way your physical calm overcomes the small amount of anxiety that you feel as you approach the dreaded situation step by step. Following are some instructions for desensitizing yourself to a fear-producing situation, then an example. *Keep in mind that if your discomfort increases as you try this method, or if you experience no change and find your anxiety worsening, you should stop the exercise and consider seeking professional help instead. Many people are able to use these methods on their own, but for some people and in some circumstances professional guidance is desirable and more effective.*

1. Make a list of different parts or versions of the situation that make you feel uncomfortable. Arrange these elements into scenes that you can imagine in very vivid detail and put the scenes in order so that the least difficult ones come first. Your list should include 10 to 20 scenes. To help yourself arrange them in order, rate each scene on a discomfort scale of 0 to 100, on which 0 means the scene creates no discomfort whatsoever and 100 means you have almost unbearable discomfort just thinking about it.

Ideally your scenes should be evenly spaced on this "discomfort thermometer."

2. Write each scene on an index card and then put the cards in order, beginning with the lowest discomfort score.

3. Go through the progressive deep muscle relaxation procedure as described in Chapter 18.

4. While remaining very relaxed, close your eyes and imagine the first (easiest) scene as vividly as possible. Place yourself mentally right in the situation—imagine what you would see, hear, and so forth.

5. If you feel tension building up at all, stop imagining the scene and go back to focusing on muscular relaxation. Your goal is to be able to imagine the scene with no discomfort whatsoever. When you are able to picture the scene twice for at least 20 seconds each time without feeling any tension, you are ready to go on to the next card. This may require three to seven repetitions of the same scene.

6. Continue through your list until you can vividly imagine the most difficult items without feeling tension building up.

You will probably need to break this procedure into shorter time segments, working on only a few items per session. When you start a new session, begin with the scene you were last able to visualize without feeling any discomfort. Remember, this is not an endurance test. If you feel any discomfort, switch the scene off and go back to relaxing. When you finish a session, be sure to end it with a success—the last scene you picture should be one for which you are totally relaxed.

Rod had an important job interview coming up. He knew that he tended to be quite nervous in that type of situation, and to try to deal with the nervousness he would drink more than he wanted to. He decided that this time he would try something else. He used the systematic desensitization instructions and prepared the following sequence of scenes 2 weeks before the actual interview:

Situation	*Discomfort Score*
1. *Thinking about the day 1 week before the actual interview.*	10
2. *Thinking about the night before the actual interview.*	30
3. *Imagining breakfast on the day of the interview.*	40
4. *Picturing myself on the day of the interview.*	45

5. *I am entering the building.*	*55*
6. *I am sitting in the waiting room.*	*65*
7. *I am being asked to come in.*	*70*
8. *I am asked the first question.*	*80*
9. *I am in the middle of the interview.*	*85*
10. *I make a dumb mistake during the interview.*	*95*

Rod set aside 20 minutes each weekday to work on this list of scenes. He found that the first few items went by fairly easily, but the higher ones took a bit longer. He made sure that he was very deeply relaxed before he started to imagine each scene, and he stopped imagining it if he felt either the queasy feeling in the pit of his stomach that was the first sign of anxiety for him or the desire to pour himself a drink. He mastered the last items just 4 days before the interview, and he continued to go over them once a day after that. Unlike other times, the night before the interview Rod chose not to drink. On the day of the interview he felt much calmer than he had expected. During the actual interview he did make a mistake in explaining a project that he had worked on, but he didn't get rattled and was able to correct himself quickly. The interview went smoothly, and as Rod was leaving he realized that, whether or not he got the job, he had presented himself well. Again, unlike other times, he did not make a beeline for the nearest bar. Instead he took his wife out to dinner.

There are several variations on the basic desensitization procedure. Two particularly useful ones are coping desensitization and live desensitization.

Coping Desensitization

This variation takes into account the fact that sometimes one cannot leave fearful situations as easily as one can stop imagining them. It focuses on learning to *cope* with a stressful situation by relaxing away tension. This is done first in the imagination, as a step toward learning to do so in reality.

Here is the variation: instead of switching off the image when it produces discomfort, maintain the image in your mind's eye. Imagine yourself coping effectively with the situation and at the same time try to relax away the tension by using your progressive muscle relaxation skills. This is how you might deal with the situation in real life, and this method provides practice in preparation for the real thing. It also helps you identify early feelings of tension and use these feelings as a signal for starting to relax. The gradual approach—starting with the easiest and working up to the most difficult scenes—is still very important.

Every other aspect of the desensitization procedure remains the same. The only difference is that in standard desensitization you are to imagine scenes without starting to feel tension, whereas in coping desensitization you are to actively reduce tension produced by each scene. Before you advance to a more difficult scene, you should be able to relax away all tension while imagining previous scenes.

Live Desensitization

Either standard or coping desensitization procedures can be applied using the actual objects or situations instead of imagined scenes. When actual situations or objects are used, it is called live, or *in vivo*, desensitization.

The difference here is that you arrange a series of real-life situations in order of their difficulty. If you are afraid of heights, you might arrange to look out of windows on the first, second, third, fourth, and fifth floors of a building, or you might arrange to look out of a high window for 30 seconds, 60 seconds, 2 minutes, 5 minutes, and so on. You may be able to use the same scenes that you would use in your imagination.

To use the standard method in live situations, relax deeply and then place yourself in the least distressing situation on your list. If you feel tension mounting, withdraw from the situation and go somewhere to become relaxed again. Once relaxed, return to the scene and repeat the procedure until you can remain in the situation comfortably for a reasonable period of time. (What is a reasonable period of time will vary according to the situation in question.) When you have mastered one situation, go on to the next most difficult one.

To use coping desensitization in real-life situations, begin by relaxing yourself as completely as you can. Then place yourself in the least distressing situation on your list. If you begin to feel tense, do not withdraw but rather try to relax away all tension until you feel comfortable once again. When you succeed in this, go on to the next most difficult situation.

Exposure and Response Prevention Therapy

More recent approaches to anxiety have focused on exposing the person who suffers from anxiety to the feared event or object and helping the person stay in the situation to learn that the fear or panic associated with the event or object eventually passes without triggering negative outcomes. Eventually, the fear is no longer triggered by the event or the object. For relatively moderate anxiety responses, it may be helpful to try this approach, which is a variation of the live desensitization method described above. For severe anxiety, we recommend seeking a therapist who specializes in cognitive-behavioral therapy for anxiety. Exposure and response prevention therapy is one of the methods used by cognitive-behavioral therapists.

Acceptance and Commitment Therapy

A relatively recent form of therapy, named acceptance and commitment therapy (ACT), emphasizes the potential negative aspects of struggling desperately to change thoughts or behaviors that are painful and the benefits of mindfully noticing their reality and, rather than focusing on them, committing oneself to acting according to one's values. There have been many studies that show that this approach is helpful for several problems.

Some Tips for the Use of Desensitization

Each of these variations is better suited to certain kinds of situations. If you're afraid of spiders, for example, it may be difficult to collect enough spiders to do live desensitization. Using your imagination would probably be more practical in this case. On the other hand, the live method might be better for a fear of leaving the house. You could gradually increase your distance from the door or your time away from home.

Once you become familiar with the principles involved, you can combine different versions to suit your situation. For example, you could practice some desensitization items in your imagination, some items using coping desensitization, and some items using live desensitization. Practice the standard method as described at the beginning of the chapter before trying out the variations. And remember: Be systematic!

A final tip on the technique of desensitization: When making your list of distressing scenes, remember that you can vary the discomfort produced by the same object or situation by changing some of its elements, such as size, length of time, distance from you, number of people involved, and so forth. It is very easy to produce any of these changes in your imagination. Use this tip to come up with more evenly spaced scenes (based on each item's discomfort score) for your lists.

Dealing with Unpleasant Memories

We all have memories that make us wince because they are embarrassing, as well as memories that make us sad or anxious. When people learn to deal with these unpleasant memories by drinking, they set themselves up to become dependent on alcohol to handle such memories. The old phrase about "drinking to forget" actually fits these people. Unfortunately, until they actually learn to deal with these memories in other ways, the memories will continue to hound them and continue to make them uncomfortable. One way to stop memories from forcing you to drink is to find alternative ways for managing them.

Systematic desensitization may be used to ease painful memories. Arrange parts of the memory in a list, from least to most disturbing element. Desensitize yourself to the list as explained in the previous sections, until the emotional impact of the memory is brought down to a neutral level. We also found desensitization to be an effective way to resolve recurrent nightmares.

If the methods we've described so far don't appeal to you, consider the following alternatives for dealing with unpleasant or unresolved memories:

1. Get it off your chest by telling it to someone you trust. Just hearing yourself talk about it sometimes helps you digest it and work it through. You can ask your friend to just listen, being understanding but not giving any advice or opinion.

2. Write it down. Getting it all down on paper where you can see it sometimes helps to make the memory more manageable. Set aside a block of time to do this. Write down the full memory and all that you feel: good feelings, bad feelings, hopes and fears, doubts and certainties. If the memory has to do with a particular person, you may want to write your thoughts in letter form. You can decide later whether or not to mail the letter. The value is usually in the writing, not in the mailing of it.

3. Set aside certain times just to think about the memory. During this reserved time, do nothing but think about the memory. Don't distract yourself with work, recreation, eating, or drinking. Just sit and think. During the rest of the day, put the memory away. If the memory intrudes, imagine yourself yelling the word "Stop!" This breaks the chain of thought. (It sounds too simple, but try it!) Or merely tell yourself: "I will devote time to this memory later in the day." The idea behind this approach is that, by controlling when the memory occurs, you can begin to feel mastery over it, and its emotional charge may diminish.

4. Experiment with "reshaping" the idea. If the way you think about a past event continually brings about emotional pain, you might be able to think about the idea in other ways. It can help to conceive of the idea as though it were a physical object that can be turned over, dismantled, or even discarded.

A key point in dealing with difficult memories or, more generally, with difficult thoughts, is to remember that thoughts are temporary events in the brain. They are not always accurate, or even if accurate they may not be relevant to our current circumstances. It may not be necessary to give them much attention or even any attention at all. Thoughts are not always faithful reflections of reality. They can be distorted by emotions, for example. And even if they are accurate, they may still be both unnecessary and harmful. If you think of thoughts as objects, in this case mental objects, you can learn to work with them so that they don't cause you unnecessary suffering. Ideas, thoughts, or memories can be useful tools and are clearly constant companions in your internal world, your internal reality. It can be useful to ask yourself whether specific thoughts pollute your internal environment and whether other thoughts bring light, life, and health to your mental universe. This way of thinking can increase your power over your thoughts and decrease the power they have over your feelings.

Thoughts are temporary events in the brain and may not be accurate, relevant, or deserving of attention in the current situation. Don't believe everything you think!

One of our clients had lost her teenage son in a particularly painful and gruesome manner. She had been unable to proceed with her life for several years, and both she and her family (she had other children) were being affected severely by her emotional state and by her excessive use of alcohol to deal with the painful memory, over and above the obvious trauma of the young man's loss. This was obviously a very difficult and delicate case. It was important to help the woman go on with her life without trivializing what had happened. She needed to be able to remember her son without being incapacitated by the memory.

At one of our sessions we commented that her son's life had lasted 17 years and was thus much longer than the moment of his death. We described his life as a 17-year-long line and likened the line to a handheld telescope. She was remembering his life as though she were looking through one of the lenses of the telescope, namely the day of his death, and thus her eyes were brimming with images of his suffering and the horrible manner in which he had died. By looking at his whole life through this lens, she could not see any other part of his life except through the pain of his last moments. Then we suggested that she mentally take the telescope and turn it so she could see it from the side and notice its length. Then we asked her to similarly "see" her son's life in its totality.

Something clicked in her at that moment, and, for the first time in therapy, she began to smile and to recall how he had been a practical joker (something she had never mentioned before). She began to chuckle at remembering some of the things her son had done. This relatively simple mental exercise was enough to provide her with noticeable relief. Therapy continued for some time thereafter, but this session and this mental exercise represented a key moment in her progress.

In this chapter we've presented many ways of managing one aspect of your internal reality, anxiety and fear, without the use of alcohol. The desensitization methods directly address the feelings of anxiety and systematically reduce the intensity of your reaction by exposing you to gradually more difficult situations. The other methods involve becoming aware of thoughts as "things" that have a harmful or helpful impact on you and learning how to respond to the thoughts in ways that bring them more under your control instead of the other way around.

All of these methods can be quite useful via self-help. But it's important to understand that anxiety and fears can reach severe proportions that require professional help. As we mentioned earlier in the chapter, if your anxiety and fear are interfering with your life or activities a lot, you should seek help from a professional rather than trying to resolve the problems on your own. For example, if you're finding it difficult to leave home to go to work or school, or to drive, or to talk with others, and you've tried the ideas in this or other books without success, it's time to consult a mental health professional. Alcohol is not helpful in this case and may in fact exacerbate the problem by increasing the chances that you will become at least psychologically dependent on it.

26

•

Being Assertive

Marcia was easy to intimidate. And she knew that about herself. So when she changed jobs, she decided she would also change her reputation and let her new coworkers know she could stand up for herself. She had always heard that a drink could give one a little extra courage, so when she was going to have a tough meeting in the afternoon, she began to have a drink with lunch. She found that the drink did relax her a bit and that she could sometimes be more forceful in making her arguments. But there was some unpredictability about the alcohol: Sometimes she actually became a bit louder than necessary. Sometimes she became a bit confused about her facts. And when she had to schedule difficult meetings in the morning, she was in trouble. She did not want to begin drinking before work, yet she felt quite overwhelmed without the help of the alcohol. The result was that rather than developing a reputation as a pushover, she was developing a reputation of being unpredictable and moody.

What does assertiveness have to do with drinking? Frustration and anger are common results of ineffective coping and are also common triggers for drinking. Good assertive communication can help you refuse unwanted (or even wanted) drinks, help you say what you want to say without the use of alcohol to bolster your courage, and help you avoid the kind of frustration and bottling up of feelings that sometimes leads to "needing" a drink.

Sometimes people drink just to please friends who insist they drink.

Perhaps you use alcohol at times because it makes it seem easier to express anger or disapproval, to stick up for your rights, to express approval or affection, to act in ways that are usually frowned on, or to express your opinions. Sometimes people drink just to please friends who insist they drink. A person with the ability to be assertive does not need alcohol to cope with feelings and situations such as these.

Assertive, Aggressive, and Passive Behavior

"Being assertive" means acting in a firm but not overly aggressive manner. It means respecting the rights and desires of others, but not to the point at which you passively allow them to trample over your own rights and needs.

Assertiveness is a middle road between the two extremes of being too aggressive and too passive.

Learning how to be assertive is important. Some people insist on their own way and become quite *aggressive* in demanding it, hurting or offending those around them. Other people never learn to be assertive and instead remain quite *passive*. Both of these are extremes, often learned while growing up. Assertiveness is a middle road between the two extremes of being too aggressive and too passive.

Aggressive people push too hard. They attempt to get their way by pushing other people around. They may raise their voice, even shout, call names, or be much too demanding, never willing to compromise. The ironic thing is that this kind of behavior often results, in the long run, in frustration and alienation. By going overboard and being too demanding, an aggressive person loses both cooperation and friendships.

Passive people, on the other hand, allow others to determine what's going to happen. They don't express their own feelings and desires and therefore seldom achieve what they want. They feel weak and frustrated.

Assertiveness involves telling people what you really feel but in a diplomatic way, especially when you are saying something that can affect what's about to happen. If you're being offered a drink, for example, and you've decided not to drink any more that night, an assertive response would be to tell the person that you don't want the drink. You might say,

> "No, thank you!"
> "I'm fine, thanks!"
> "I'd enjoy another one, but I've decided not to."

Or, if the other person insists,

> "Please don't insist. I said no."

These would be assertive responses. An aggressive response would be to get angry and snap back. A passive response would be to accept the drink and drink it.

Some types of situations that call for some skill in assertiveness are:

- Telling someone that you like him or like what he did.
- Telling someone that you disapprove of what she did.
- Asking someone to do a favor for you.
- Telling someone that you don't want to do what she has asked.

How aggressive or passive are you? Ask yourself:

- Do I pride myself on being "forceful"?
- Do I tend to raise my voice when in a difficult situation?
- Have I shouted when I was not getting my way?
- Do I bully my way through situations?
- Do I try to frighten people into doing things my way?
- Do I blow up when things don't go the way I want them to?

If you're answering "yes," chances are you're being too aggressive.

- Do I keep quiet and let whatever happens happen?
- Am I afraid to tell people what I like or think?
- Do I go ahead and do what others decide, even though it may not meet my needs?
- Do I often regret not having told people what I really wanted to do?
- Do I often find myself resenting doing things other people wanted because I didn't speak up and say I didn't want to do that?
- Do I often find myself replaying a situation in my head, wishing I had been more forceful?

If you're answering "yes" to these questions, you're probably being too passive. To increase your assertiveness, here are four steps that may help:

1. Identify times and places at which you could be assertive but usually are not.

2. Notice how other people handle these situations. Find people who act assertively (firm but not overly aggressive). Study what they do. Pay attention to specific words and gestures.

3. Practice being assertive. Start by practicing mentally, that is, in your internal world. Use your imagination to the fullest. Imagine exactly what you might do. Sit down in a quiet place, close your eyes, and start

imagining the scene. Imagine the place. Imagine yourself and the other people involved. Then start the action. You want to see yourself acting assertively. Imitate what the assertive people you've seen would do in this situation. Change their words and gestures so that you're comfortable, but don't lose the assertive quality in them. Be very specific in picturing yourself being assertive. Instruct yourself to "keep eye contact" or to "speak clearly," for example. Picture yourself actually going through the actions. Finally, imagine yourself feeling good about having been assertive. Notice how good it feels to have told someone what you wanted to say. Think how frustrated you would have felt if you had not expressed yourself. Or think how much more negatively others would have reacted if you had blown your top. Practice until you can go through it smoothly in your imagination. Then try it out in actual situations.

4. Keep track of your progress in an assertiveness diary. When you try new assertive behaviors, write down what you did, how it worked, and how you felt. It's a good way to remind yourself how you're doing.

Expressing Negative Feelings and Positive Feelings

When you express negative feelings, concentrate on being polite but firm. If you're uncomfortable with someone's behavior, it's usually OK to let the person know in very clear terms. This does not mean that you need to insult or intimidate the other person. If you do, the person may become defensive, making it harder for you to achieve your objective. A good test is to imagine how you would prefer to be told something negative, so that you would understand the person's feelings but would not feel threatened or humiliated. When you have a good picture of that situation, try it out.

It's also OK, under most circumstances, to let people know your positive feelings. If you like what someone has done, for example, you can say so without hesitation. You have every right to do so, and most people enjoy hearing compliments even if they become a bit self-conscious. Again, try to imagine how you would like someone else to tell you something positive, then try doing it that way.

So, What Do You Say?

Some people find that they get stuck in trying to come up with assertive responses when it comes to deciding exactly what words to use. There are many different ways of saying the same thing effectively. The exact words are not as important as getting the message across clearly. Nevertheless, you do need words to use, and it's a good idea to plan exactly how you might say something in an assertive manner. Here are some examples of assertive statements:

"Please don't smoke. It really bothers me."

"This is the third time you've been late, and that annoys me."

"It feels great being here with you."

"Good job!"

"No, thanks. I've had just enough to feel good, and any more would spoil it."

"I need a hand with this. Can you help me, please?"

"I really can't afford the time to help you until next week."

"I don't like being called 'Honey'!"

"I really enjoyed that dessert."

"That movie doesn't interest me."

"Sunday is a bad night for me. How about Friday or Saturday instead?"

"No, I don't think I should give you any more to drink. You have to drive home, and I'd feel terrible if anything happened to you because I gave you too much."

"You handled that beautifully."

"I am very angry with you."

"I want to talk to you about something that's been on my mind."

"Excuse me. I was here first."

"Please give me another package. This one has been opened."

Assertiveness in Action

To help you begin thinking about situations in which assertiveness can be useful, here are some examples.

• You're visiting relatives, and your uncle Bob begins his usual inquiry about when you're going to get "a decent job." You're tired of having to justify yourself to him and the rest of your family, and you know that if the conversation continues you'll become angry.

UNCLE BOB: "Well, when are you going to settle into a decent job? Any prospects yet?"

YOU: "Uncle Bob, I know you care about me, but I'd really rather you didn't ask me about my job every time we talk. Let's talk about something else and enjoy being together, OK?"

• You are single and have just gone out with someone for the first time. You really enjoyed yourself but find it hard to say so. In this case, telling the person how good you feel would be an assertive act. It need not be a magnificent statement. It need only convey the message "I enjoyed being with you." You could use these words or be more specific about what you did enjoy:

"I really enjoyed dancing with you tonight."
"This was a really relaxing afternoon. You're fun to be with."
"I enjoyed talking to you. You have a lot of interesting ideas."
"It was fun talking to someone who is as interested in music as I am."

• Your best friend is pushing drinks on someone who you know is trying to cut down. You're annoyed at your friend and think she isn't being fair. An assertive response here might involve taking your friend aside and saying, "Hey, I wonder if you realize that Sam is trying to cut down on his drinking. He's having a hard time, and it's even harder when people push drinks on him. How about helping him out?"

• A salesperson calls you on the phone and asks for a few minutes of your time. You could afford the time but really don't want to buy anything. Besides, you dislike sales talk. The salesperson says, "Just let me describe our offer, no obligation. If you don't find our offer beneficial, you haven't lost anything." One assertive response would be "No, thank you. I'm not interested. Good-bye." You could then hang up, making your decision clear.

When Marcia came across the concept of assertiveness, she knew that's what she needed to develop and practice. But she found that part of the reason she was passive most of the time was that she did not want to hurt people's feelings. To make it easier on herself, she began analyzing situations such as the one with the salesperson to "rechannel her stream of consciousness" into a path that would make it easier to be assertive. In this case she told herself the following: "Think about it: if you're clear, not only are you saving your time, but you're also saving the salesperson's time because you weren't going to buy anything anyway." That thought made it easier to be clear-cut and brief.

27

·

Relating to Others

Walking into a party was the hardest thing for Carla. It was worst when she didn't know the people, but even when she did she found herself unable to start a conversation. So she would make a beeline for the drinks, pour herself one, and gulp it down as soon as possible. Within a few minutes the edges of things around her became a bit softer, her anxiety was less noticeable, and she didn't care as much what others would think. She had been doing this since high school, and she figured she would need to keep doing it indefinitely.

One reason that people sometimes give for drinking is that it helps them become more sociable—to meet, be friendly with, and become closer to other people. The use of alcohol to facilitate sociability is common in our society and is fairly well accepted. It's when you have no alternative to alcohol that this becomes a potential problem. You've probably heard the line "If you need a drink to be social, that's not social drinking."

Sometimes alcohol becomes a problem for people who have a hard time meeting other people and starting ongoing relationships. This can occur as a result of shyness or isolation, perhaps due to having moved to a new community or having left a particularly supportive group of friends and family. However, sometimes this could be the result of severe social anxiety. If the suggestions in this chapter are relevant to your drinking patterns, but are not enough to help you develop more social connections, you may want to consider obtaining professional help. Social contacts contribute to having a healthy life. They are worth paying attention to if you are feeling so isolated that the loneliness becomes emotionally painful.

If you need a drink to be social, that's not social drinking.

Forming Relationships

As society becomes increasingly mobile, it becomes more important to be able to start relationships with a variety of people. When you're separated from your family and friends, you need to establish new relationships. And it's always important to get along well with supervisors, colleagues, and subordinates at work. Some people find it easy to start relationships; others do not. If you are one who does not, you might find yourself feeling isolated and also increasingly anxious about connecting with new people. These feelings can lead some people to drink to "loosen up," as with Carla. If forming relationships is a problem for you, there are ways to get over the hump without alcohol.

There are at least four steps involved in forming new relationships. Each step requires different personal skills.

Finding People

If you're not around other people, you can't meet them. It's important to find situations in which you're likely to talk with new people. The more assertive you are (Chapter 26), the easier this will be. You can, however, increase the chances of your meeting and talking with someone interesting by doing a little planning. A good general rule to make new friends is:

Do what you find interesting, but do it in the company of other people.

Find a class or a club or a group in which you can do what you enjoy with others rather than doing it alone. This has at least two advantages. First of all, you're most interesting when you're involved in things that you enjoy and do well. Second, you're most likely to meet people with similar interests when you're in such groups.

Volumes have been written about the effects of social networking, and the debate about whether Internet platforms improve or detract from interpersonal relationships and social skills continues. Issues of privacy and security aside, adults have an opportunity to connect with those of like mind or interests like never before, thanks to online chat rooms, forums, blogs, message boards, and networking sites like Facebook, LinkedIn, and Myspace. If you can use these outlets to expand your social circle, they offer a great opportunity not only to connect but also to polish your communication skills. The key, naturally, is not to substitute virtual connections for all in-person relationships.

Do what you find interesting, but do it in the company of other people.

Meeting People

Once you've picked out the places where you're most likely to be around people you could meet and with whom you may share some common interests, make it a point to go there often. The more comfortable you feel in a situation, the more familiar you become with the social rules of a place, and the easier it is to interact with others. You could help to orient newcomers, for example. If you're having difficulty feeling comfortable in social situations, try progressive relaxation and desensitization (Chapters 18 and 25). This is also a good time to use assertiveness skills (Chapter 26).

Becoming Acquainted

This involves making arrangements to see people in other situations. You may have to take the first step to begin getting acquainted with someone, and this is another situation in which assertiveness helps. Of course, not every acquaintance is likely to become a friend.

Maintaining and Deepening a Relationship

The skills involved in developing close personal relationships are too complex to summarize here, but there are some general guidelines:

- Be honest about your feelings, both with yourself and with the other person.
- Pay attention to the other person. Listen. Be sincerely interested in what she or he has to say and how he or she sees things. "Taking for granted" has to do with forgetting to pay attention to the other.
- Communicate clearly what you like and do not like.
- Remember that a good relationship requires the investment of time and effort. Set aside time that is devoted exclusively to your relationship—for talking, playing, sharing, caring.
- Don't set unrealistic expectations for yourself, for the other person, or for your relationship. No one else can fulfill all or even most of your needs.

One of the things that prompted Carla to read about how to become more sociable (without using alcohol) was that she began to feel the need to develop a serious relationship. And she wanted to be able to talk with potential romantic partners while her mind was clear. Also, she wanted to find a partner who was comfortable either drinking or not drinking. After dating several guys, she found Matt. He was really special. He had no trouble expressing his affection for her, and she loved making him feel loved. However, after several months she became quite frightened about a sudden change in her feelings: the strong attraction she felt seemed to fade away. He was still affectionate and romantic, but she no longer felt the "head over heels" magic she had felt until then. This is when she began having trouble with her drinking. She was surprised at the fact that it was her sudden ambivalence that caused her so much stress. She would have understood it if he had suddenly turned cold toward her, if she had felt rejected. But what bothered her was the fluctuation of her own feelings toward Matt. And, when they were together socially, she found herself drinking more than usual. It was as if she wanted to deaden the discomfort she felt being with Matt without the strong romantic attraction she had felt at first. She wondered whether the fact that her feelings had changed was a sign that Matt was not the right man for her or whether it meant that there was something wrong with her, that she was fickle and unfair to him. Matt, of course, noticed the change and began to worry about her increased drinking. And, when he began to show signs of considering cooling off the relationship, Carla surprisingly (though perhaps predictably as well) felt her anxiety go through the roof. She was afraid of losing him.

Learning from Others

If you feel awkward or shy around others, and that has kept you from pursuing relationships, it might help to learn from other people who seem to navigate social waters with ease. If you feel like you tend to put your foot in your mouth or you somehow end up in conflicts where you never intended to, others' communication skills can serve as good models. We go into handling conflicts below; there are also many excellent books on the subject of communicating in relationships, from workplace relationships to intimate partnerships.

Observe and learn from socially skilled persons.

Think of people you know who are good at meeting and becoming friends with others. Observe what they do around others. Of course it looks easy for them to do it. No effort seems to be involved, and you're tempted to think that they were born with social graces. But that's just because they've learned their social skills well enough to put them into practice quite comfortably. Think of an athlete and how easy he or she makes those astonishing moves look.

Observe and learn from socially skilled persons. Make two different kinds of observations:

1. Observe specific behaviors. You will, for example, probably find that people who are "understanding" and "sociable" do the following:

   - *Smile* from time to time. When do they smile? How much and how often?
   - *Keep eye contact* at a comfortable level. Notice that most people who are seen as "understanding" often look the other person in the eye when listening. (This varies greatly across cultures, by the way.)
   - *Show that they are listening.* Good listeners show this by nodding, saying "mm-hmm," rephrasing what the speaker said to make sure they understand, offering relevant experiences from their own lives, or showing agreement with comments such as "That's right!" and "I know what you mean" and "I feel the same way sometimes."

2. Observe the tone and meaning of the interaction. You will probably find that understanding people:

   - *Maintain attentiveness* and are genuinely interested in the other person
   - Show *respect* for the other
   - *Rarely criticize*
   - *Don't give advice* unless asked
   - Are not *possessive* or "*pushy*"
   - *Don't tell people what to do*
   - *Pay attention* to the other person's feelings
   - *Match the other's level of seriousness* (not making jokes when the other person wants to be serious and not taking things too seriously when the other person is being humorous)
   - *Make the other person feel at ease*
   - *Don't whine or complain*

Both kinds of observation are important, and they are related. As you observe the overall tone of the interaction, try to understand just what the understanding person is doing to set that tone. As you discover the skillful behaviors of others, put them together in a way that fits your own style.

> *To deal with her anxiety, Carla joined a support group for women. The group was diverse in many ways, including age. She gravitated toward Rebecca, an older woman who seemed very wise to her. Rebecca was going through mourning for her husband of 40 years. One evening, during the group meeting, Rebecca shared an insight that was very helpful to Carla. She recounted how she had been involved with another man before she married her husband and how much in love she had felt at first. She then went through a period in which her feelings for this man cooled off, and she decided to call off their relationship. When she started her relationship with her husband, the same thing happened, and again, she considered ending the relationship. But one day the following thought came to her: Feelings toward loved ones do fluctuate. She didn't feel the same level of affection toward her mother or her brother all the time. In fact, even her feelings about herself fluctuated: Sometimes she liked herself better than at other times. Sometimes she was even irritated with herself. It was probably unrealistic, then, to expect that romantic feelings would remain at the same level of intensity all the time. Once she had this insight, she felt less anxious, and was able to open herself enough to consider whether she was still romantically attracted to him, whether she respected and trusted him enough to want to marry him, and whether she felt he loved her as well. She was able to experience the ups and downs of passion, the moments of doubt or irritation, the moments of peace and bliss, and finally decided that this was the man she wanted to build a life with. She now missed him terribly, but she was very happy that they had shared the time they had had. Rebecca's experience was helpful to Carla because it pointed out to her that emotions do fluctuate and that her decision of whether to pursue her relationship with a potential partner needed to be made on the basis of many factors, not just her current (and changeable) level of attraction. She realized that making a final decision about Matt would be more complicated than ending the relationship because she was feeling some doubts.*

When Conflicts Arise in Close Relationships

For two or more people to live together in harmony there must be a continual give and take—a kind of compromising. Often this happens naturally, without much awareness. At times, however, one or another person becomes dissatisfied with the result of this natural process and conflict arises.

Often people are able to come up with an acceptable solution to a problem by talking it over and arriving at an understanding. This requires attention to each other's needs and wants. Sometimes, however, talking does not produce the needed changes, and a more systematic kind of solution process is needed, a process of negotiation.

Negotiation is a method for dealing with problems between people who are close to each other. It is a method that permits people to respect and understand each other while arranging for their own needs to be met. Here is a brief outline of how the process works.

1. When a conflict arises in a relationship, set a time to talk it over. Put aside a period of time that is reserved solely for solving the problem. Negotiation deserves your full attention. Arrange a time and place where you won't be interrupted. Once you've agreed on a time to discuss it, don't waste time rehashing the conflict before your negotiation session.

2. Commit yourself to seeking a constructive and mutually satisfying "win–win" solution to the problem. Think of the problem as something

Statements that begin with "You do this or that" sound very accusatory.

that is neither inside you nor inside the other person but that is affecting you both. Avoid unfair and provocative actions, such as making insulting remarks, threatening, blaming, and bringing up old complaints. Stay focused on the *problem* you've agreed to discuss, not on whether either of you is to blame. Talk over only one problem at a time.

3. Begin by getting a clear picture of the conflict. Each person could write down the *specific behavior* that he or she sees as being the problem. For example:

"You don't pay the bills on time as we agreed you would."
"You tie up the bathroom for half an hour in the morning."

This is difficult. Be careful to avoid general name-calling complaints that only sound like the problem:

Too general: "You're inconsiderate."
Better: "Please call when you're going to be late."
Too general: "You're sloppy."
Better: "I feel irritated when you leave your work on the kitchen table."

Note that statements that begin with "You do this or that" sound very accusatory. Statements that focus on what you feel or prefer are less provocative.

4. Clearly specify what changes are needed. If you have carefully specified the problem in Step 3, this is much easier. For example:

> "If you'll put the mail here on the desk, I'll check for bills every day and make sure they're paid on time."
> "I will spend no more than 20 minutes in the bathroom in the morning."

Negotiations tend to have a more balanced feeling if each partner ends up with one change to be made. Remember that it is absolutely essential that the change be specified clearly. It should be obvious to a neutral observer when the change has been made and when it has not.

5. When the other person makes a change in behavior as requested, notice and comment positively on it. Consider doing something nice as a "thank you."

If negotiating fails to ease your conflicts, consider seeking some professional counseling. A neutral third perspective can be helpful, and many psychologists and other professionals have special training and experience in dealing with relationship problems. Consider seeking outside assistance if you cannot reach mutually satisfying solutions, if you cannot negotiate without becoming embroiled in argument, or if conflicts escalate toward physical violence.

> *When Matt complained to Carla that she had been drinking more than he was comfortable with, she acknowledged that that was the case and asked if he would be willing to sit down and talk about what was troubling her. They set up a time and drove to a place overlooking the ocean, where they could talk without interruptions. He let her know that he was upset because she appeared to be withdrawing emotionally and seemed to be comfortable with him only when she was drinking. He was starting to think that unless she was drinking she was not enjoying his company. This was different from the way it had been for the first few months they were together. She had decided that, for the relationship to have a chance of becoming lifelong, it would have to withstand even the sharing of doubts about itself. She swallowed hard and told him about her ambivalence and her fluctuating feelings.*

Matt was quiet for a while. When he finally talked, his tone had gone back to the way it was when they first expressed their caring for each other. He was sad to hear that her ardor had cooled, but he was willing to give her the time she needed to decide. He was sure he wanted to continue the relationship, but he didn't want Carla to be with him if she didn't want him. One thing that he was clear on was that her excessive drinking was turning him off. He needed to know that she would go back to the way it had been when they first met. "Relationships are hard enough to manage without adding the complications of too much alcohol to the mix," he said.

She agreed and asked him to remind her of their agreement if she seemed to have forgotten it. He thanked her for trusting him enough to tell him what she was feeling. She thanked him for being understanding. They hugged for a long time, looking out at the ocean, both wondering where their future would lead.

28

•

Living "As If"

Leo had been the class clown since grammar school. In high school, one of his favorite tricks was pretending he was roaring drunk. In college, he began drinking heavily, until being drunk was no longer an act. After college, he was able to get a job he really wanted, which had a lot of potential for advancement. He decided that he no longer wanted to drink to the point of being drunk. By this time, however, he found it difficult to enjoy himself in social situations without using alcohol. And once he began drinking, it was hard for him to control how much he drank. When he started the self-control program, it occurred to him that using his old "acting" skills might come in handy. After all, he had been really good at acting as if he was totally drunk. He could act as if he had had enough alcohol to loosen up and enjoy himself in a way that fit with the new image he was trying to live up to: friendly without being intrusive, happy without being obnoxious, spontaneous without being totally unpredictable. It took several tries to get just the right level he wanted, but once he hit his stride, he was the spitting image of the charming social drinker. And once he developed confidence that he could behave the way he wanted, he found it easier to limit his number of drinks: he no longer needed them to feel at ease.

Acting "As If"

We believe that people have a remarkable ability to change themselves, as well as a remarkable ambivalence about doing so. Those who learn the ability to act "as if" have the freedom to experiment with other ways of acting and feeling—to try out how it would feel to be a different kind of person. The ability to act "as if" is the ability to step out of one role or behavior and into another.

Actors are people who have the ability to step into the role of someone they are not. They can perform those roles in a very convincing manner. When you're watching an effective actor, you see not the actor but rather the person being portrayed. Actors who have played the same role again and again even report beginning to feel like the person they've been playing.

All of us have a certain amount of acting ability, and it can be used to good advantage. For example, have you ever wished you were

More sociable?
Friendlier?
Wittier?
Able to let go and loosen up?
Able to blend in better with other people?
Able to really enjoy yourself?
More entertaining?
In a better mood?

What would happen if you temporarily took on the role you wished for? It can be done. You can use this method to shape yourself—internally and externally. In this way you can begin to shape your personal reality, starting with your mind and behavior.

1. You need to know how a person looks and acts who has the quality you desire. Suppose you wish to be a more sociable person. You first need to know what sociable people act like. This is the equivalent of an actor studying the character to be portrayed.
2. Practice acting that way. Do the kinds of things that "sociable" people do. This is the equivalent of rehearsing for a performance.
3. Get ready for your grand opening. Select a day and tell yourself, "On that day I am going to try out being a sociable person." Think about how a sociable person feels. This is the equivalent of "getting into the role."
4. Do it! Try out your new role. It's only an experiment, after all. Do sociable things all day or for a particular period of time. Act like a sociable person.
5. Think about it. Did people respond differently to you? How did you feel? Decide whether you would like to be more like that every

day. Like an actor, if you play the role often enough, you begin to become the role, and the role becomes you.

People sometimes rely on alcohol to give them a boost toward many different abilities and characteristics that they don't feel come naturally to them. Being outgoing and garrulous is only one common one. You may have come to believe over time that it's only through drinking that you can transform yourself into someone who is confident, assertive, laid back, flirtatious, witty, eloquent, or a good dancer. Maybe you wish to become a different person not just socially but at work, with your spouse, or in the pursuit of some avocation, such as acting or singing or playwriting. Acting "as if" can help you become the person you aspire to in any arena. The fact is, if you didn't have the core ability to become what you desire, drinking never would have made it possible. In other words, if you are capable of acting sociably when you use alcohol, then you are capable of acting socially, period!

Acting "As If" You've Had a Drink

We'd like to suggest that you try a very interesting "as if" role. The role is one you know about. It's the role of a drinker. It's the role that Leo tried.

Many people find that when they have something to drink they feel more comfortable and act more sociable. They become more humorous, laugh more easily, can be friendlier. The result is that they enjoy themselves more than if they had not had a drink and gone through these changes.

The question is: Was it the drink or the changes in how they felt and acted that helped them enjoy themselves? If it is the changes in feeling and acting that matter, is it possible to experience them without drinking? Is it possible to act *as if* . . . ? Studies now show that people who *believe* they are drinking alcohol show many of the same changes in behavior, even if (unknown to them) their drinks do not actually contain any alcohol.

If you are capable of acting sociably when you use alcohol, then you are capable of acting sociably, period!

Many people can do a reasonable impression of a person who has had "one too many." There is the slurring of words, the precarious balance, the silly grin, the sleepy-eyed look, the embarrassing candor. You might be able to put on a good enough act to fool your friends into thinking you really are intoxicated, especially if you do it in a situation in which drinks have been freely available.

Just as you can act as if you were intoxicated, so you could imitate the way you act and feel when you've had a moderate dose of alcohol. Perhaps you stand in a certain, more relaxed way or smile more often, talk more than usual, and think less about whether or not what you're saying is proper. Perhaps you interact more with people and talk about different things. It's possible to act "as if" you've had *a few* drinks.

Try this as an experiment the next time you're with friends who are drinking. Your task will be to act as if you were drinking in your normal manner, even though you are not. (You may need to have a convincing-looking glass in your hand.) Try to imagine how you usually feel after one or two drinks and actually act it out. As the night goes on, you might even begin to act as if you've had too much to drink. You may find the role playing quite enjoyable. You may even find it hard to drop the act.

After your experiment, sit down and think about it. How did you feel? Did you get into the act? Did you enjoy yourself any more or less than usual? What did you do that made you have fun? What could you have done if you had actually been drinking that you did not do?

This is only one role you could play. There are many other possibilities. If you wish you were able to really enjoy yourself, look for people who clearly do enjoy themselves and simply emulate their behavior, whether it's going to a comedy film and laughing hard along with the rest of the audience or smiling and taking a deep breath of the morning air along with your cheerful spouse. What may feel forced at first will eventually feel natural if you stick with it. Want to be more entertaining? Watch how others do it: Maybe it's just by acting as if they're having a great time wherever they are; maybe it's by learning and telling jokes; maybe it's by showing lots of interest in those around them; maybe it's by cultivating and displaying a talent. Whatever it is, acting "as if" will open the door to potential change. The point of acting "as if" is this: By "acting" in a certain way, you're actually practicing being the person you want to be, and you can even begin to feel like that person. Experimenting with your life by acting "as if" is one way of becoming more like the person you want to be. Try it!

Some of the participants in our programs tell us they're concerned that "acting as if" feels like "faking it" and that whatever they're doing won't last because it's not genuine. From a "healthy management of reality" perspective (introduced at the beginning of Part IV), this is how we understand what's happening: When you "act as if," you're bringing two powerful forces into play. First, you're constructing a detailed picture *in your mind* of how you would think and feel if you were truly sociable, assertive, responsible, or whatever other image you wanted to project. Second, you're also systematically producing the specific *behaviors* you would undertake if you were feeling that way. The focus on the thoughts and feelings begins to change your internal reality. The focus on your actions begins to change external reality. That is, you begin to think and behave the way you want to. As you continue doing so, you're genuinely practicing this new way of being. This in turn allows you to get the rewards that sociable, assertive, and responsible people get: friendly responses, respect, and trust. The total effect is a *real* change in your mental reality (you really *are* thinking those thoughts), in your behavior (you really *are* behaving that way), and in how the external world reacts to you (people really *are* reacting to you in a new way). If you like that change, you can keep practicing the "act" until it becomes a comfortable way for you to be. When does the "act" end? When it is no longer an act.

Part V

●

How Are You Doing?

Most self-help books take a decidedly upbeat approach in the advice they give. "If you do these things, you will succeed." Consequently they often say little or nothing about what to do if you try their approach but don't succeed. At most, there may be implicit advice to "Try, try, try again"—the underlying message being that if you haven't succeeded yet, you're not following the program properly.

We are definitely *not* saying this. Although we have seen many people succeed in moderating their drinking with the methods described in this book, we have also seen many decide, after giving this program a try, to quit drinking altogether.

After you've been using the methods described in this book for 6 weeks or more, it's time to take stock of how you're doing. Are you succeeding with a goal of moderate and problem-free drinking? Don't expect perfection, but if this is going to work for you, by 6 weeks or so you should be seeing substantial progress in reducing your drinking and any related negative effects. Here are some questions to help you evaluate how you're doing with self-control of your drinking.

Yes	No	
____	____	Are you still drinking medically risky amounts of alcohol (two or more drinks a day for women or three or more drinks a day for men)?
____	____	Do you often drink more than you intended and have trouble staying within the limits you set for yourself?
____	____	Do you drive motor vehicles or do other potentially risky things while alcohol is still in your bloodstream?
____	____	Is it a struggle for you to maintain moderation, as though you were walking a tightrope and might lose your balance at any moment?
____	____	Does it seem useless or pointless to have only a drink or two?
____	____	Do you experience signs of overdrinking, such as memory impairment, injury, or poor judgment?
____	____	Are you in danger of serious negative consequences if you continue overdrinking (such as loss of family or relationship, legal consequences, job loss)?
____	____	Do you have a medical condition (such as hepatitis or stomach ulcer) that makes even moderate drinking dangerous to your health?

If you are still answering yes to one or more of these questions after giving self-control a good try, we recommend that you reevaluate. The methods described in this book are the best we know for helping people moderate their drinking on their own and constitute the only approach thus far with solid scientific evidence of effectiveness. If this isn't working for you, we recommend that you try abstaining from alcohol altogether, at least for a few months. Part V includes some specific advice if this is the path you're considering.

Chapter 29 is for those who are considering or have decided on an alcohol-free lifestyle. In it we suggest positive ways to think about abstinence and suggest some tools that have helped others who chose an alcohol-free life. Another good option is to seek support in establishing an alcohol-free life. Chapter 30 offers some guidelines in considering professional and other sources of support for sobriety.

29

•

If Moderation Isn't
Working for You

We first met Fran in Chapter 3. She had been struggling with whether to pursue moderation or abstinence and, having tried several times to stop drinking altogether without success, she decided to give this moderation program a concerted effort. As is the case with most major life choices, such decisions are the result of many factors. Fran was aware that she resented the many people who had been pushing her to quit drinking. Many of the people she knew considered this choice a religious or moral one. Fran felt as though they were trying to convert her to their faith and that this was inappropriate. As she did not share their religious or moral beliefs, why should she arrive at the same conclusion that abstinence was the only possible decision for a good person? Other people did not use religious or moral arguments, but they appeared to want her to accept that she was an "alcoholic," an image of herself that she did not share. Rather than being helpful to Fran, both of these strong perspectives actually pushed her farther from being able to make a choice to abstain, even after she realized that moderate drinking was not working for her.

When people become aware that the way they use alcohol is causing problems in their lives, one of the issues they face is how to make an independent decision about what to do. Often the pressure from others over how to drink or whether to drink at all seems like a ceaseless lecture or sermon. Pressure like this—self-righteous advice—often backfires. More often than not, it biases the person against moderation *and* abstinence. It makes people think that if they make any change in this aspect of their lives, they are capitulating to moralists, accepting the label of *alcoholic,* or bending their will to others' wishes.

This book was written to provide an alternative to the all-or-nothing approach. It is meant to counter the message that no individual who has trouble with drinking can hope to achieve moderation. It is designed to provide practical support and suggestions for those who want to attempt to establish a moderate drinking pattern. And it is based on the premise that problems concerning life and health are best addressed through scientific investigation and that individual choices are best made based on reliable data, rather than merely in response to social pressure.

Like Fran, though, you may have found moderation ineffective. Like Fran, you may feel that you've reached a dead end. You don't want to keep struggling with a method that isn't working for you; you don't want to feel like you're not in control of your own life; and you don't want to make a choice that seems like acquiescing to the view that you're a bad person if you *don't* make that choice. If so, this chapter is for you. It is intended to be of help to those who are considering an alcohol-free life. It lays out the pros and cons of drinking in the hope that you can more objectively decide for yourself whether drinking or not drinking is better for you. It is not necessary to believe that abstinence is the best lifestyle for everyone. You can merely choose not to drink.

Arguments for and against Drinking

Health, social factors, and the issue of personal freedom are considerations that most people wrestle with when trying to make decisions about whether to drink. The relative weight you assign to each of these factors and the pros and cons that are most significant to you are very personal matters, but even if you end up believing your gut instinct about whether to drink or not, you may feel better about your decision if you examine the pros and cons rationally and as objectively as possible. Use the following ideas as a start.

Health Benefits versus Health Risks

One concern that many people raise about abstaining involves the loss of the health benefits of drinking alcohol. Studies do show that people (particularly men) who drink moderately are less likely to suffer heart attacks when compared with those who do not drink at all.[24]

Although it is not completely clear that dietary alcohol is the reason for this decreased risk, it may well be. On the other hand, the risk reduction is modest, similar in size to that associated with taking an aspirin or eating a handful of nuts each day, and smaller than the benefits of moderate exercise. Furthermore, above a very moderate level of drinking (one drink a day for women and two drinks a day for men, according to the U.S. National Institutes of Health), any health benefits of alcohol are quickly overshadowed by health risks associated with heavier drinking.

So, the question to ask yourself, if you believe you're gaining a health benefit from moderate drinking, is whether you could gain the same or greater health benefit in other ways if you choose to abstain from alcohol. Could you opt for healthier eating and regular physical activity? If so, you'll also gain muscle strength, flexibility, and mood enhancement. The choice, as always, is yours. Be realistic about what you're willing and not willing to do.

As to the risks and damages, perhaps the most common reason that people give for abstaining is that they feel it is in the interest of their health. Some have learned that they are beginning to show health damage from drinking. Some have seen alcohol destroy a family member or loved one. Some have tried a short period of abstinence and just felt healthier.

One of the reasons it has been so rewarding to work with people who drink too much is that we see them get *so much better* within a relatively short span of time. In other problem areas, psychotherapy sometimes goes on for years with relatively modest change, but one doesn't need a microscope to see the changes that take place when heavy drinkers let go of alcohol. Usually they look better, feel better, are physically healthier, happier, work better, and have more rewarding relationships. This is not to say that abstinence cures all ills, only that in general things change quite a bit for the better.

As most of us are well aware, thanks to heightened attention by the news media and the diligence of our doctors, research indicates that alcohol increases the risks of many illnesses, from certain types of cancer to heart disease and many others (see Appendix A). One consideration to factor into your weighing of the health benefits and risks of alcohol for yourself, then, is the diseases for which you are already at high risk. If cancer or heart disease runs in your family or if you have other risk factors for these health problems, abstinence may be a wiser choice for you than for others. But if you don't have any of these risk factors and you're able to maintain true moderation, so that you get the health benefits of alcohol without the damage, abstinence simply boils down to a lifestyle choice for you. You don't have to have alcohol-related problems to choose not to drink. Again, the choice is yours.

Social Ease versus Social Pressure

Social pressures and other social factors are sometimes the most complicated issues to consider in a decision about whether or not to drink. Many people who drink, either moderately or heavily, do so in part because of the social ease that alcohol offers them, as well as because of social pressures to fit in. If alcohol has been a part of your life for a long time, you may not even be consciously aware of these motivations. Again, you balance the pros and cons objectively to decide whether social considerations should drive your decision to drink or to abstain.

As we discussed in Chapter 15, alcohol is not a particularly effective relaxant, but still it does help some people feel more comfortable, amicable, and confident in social settings. Sometimes the only way to determine whether the alcohol actually does promote these positive feelings is to try socializing without it. Many people find, as we've mentioned, that it's not really the drink at all that makes them feel this way; it's their expectations about what the drink will produce in them—the placebo effect—that's producing the perceived benefits.

If you think alcohol really does help you in social situations, what are the alternatives? We discussed some of them in Part IV of this book. If you have relied on alcohol to cope with certain uncomfortable situations, then finding new ways to cope gives you a choice; see Chapters 18, 21, and 27 and possibly other chapters in Part IV as well.

Another reason that people give for continuing to drink alcohol is the desire to fit in and fear of the social pressure that may be imposed if they decide not to drink anymore. Indeed, in some social situations you may feel pressure to drink or to explain or justify your choice not to do so. This is particularly true for people who have become alcohol-dependent. One thing that happens over the course of years is that heavy drinkers gravitate toward other heavy drinkers and tend to avoid nondrinking friends and social situations. After a while, it seems as though everyone drinks heavily and that abstainers must be few and far between.

Remember, however, that more than half of American adults are essentially nondrinkers (see Chapter 4), and in most cases not because they had had alcohol problems. Drinking and not drinking are individual lifestyle choices.

Still, if your circle of family and friends are mostly people who drink and encourage drinking, the decision to abstain can create other changes and challenges. The nondrinker may need to make new friends who support sobriety, providing social support for the change. It may be necessary to develop comfort with and skills for refusing drinks (see Chapters 8 and 26). If you have come to associate fun exclusively with drinking, you can discover ways to have fun and enjoy yourself with people, places, and activities that do not involve drinking. The skills described in Part IV of this book may help you find ways to enjoy life without alcohol.

If you choose to abstain, you may feel somewhat isolated from drinking friends at first, but if your decision is the right one for you, your life and lifestyle will adapt.

Even if you feel as if you're immersed in a social world in which drinking is ever present, you might find yourself getting encouragement for a decision to abstain from those close to you. Some heavy drinkers respond well to encouragement to quit from people who love them. One man turned up in our clinic "because two of my friends who don't know each other told me, in the same week, that they were worried about my drinking." Some seek treatment with pressure from their employer or the courts. Others are faced with the possible loss of intimate partners or their families if they keep on drinking. In fact, most of those who go through the doors of an alcohol treatment center are receiving some external encouragement to get help. They are the lucky ones, because it's usually those around a person who first see alcohol problems emerging, long before a drinker realizes it him- or herself. By the time people come for help strictly on their own, they have usually suffered far greater negative consequences and health damage. There's nothing wrong with deciding to make a change "for someone else," at least in the beginning.

There's nothing wrong with deciding to make a change "for someone else," at least in the beginning.

If you're thinking about choosing not to drink, you will probably start to notice, if you haven't already, how pervasive social and cultural messages are that adult (and, unfortunately, adolescent) drinking is the norm. Alcohol advertising is one omnipresent source of social pressure to drink, of course, and sometimes this pressure seems to be built into the fabric of society.

Don, a professor at a major university, encountered the following examples during the first few weeks he tried to abstain:

- At a celebration for a prominent professor at a national scientific meeting, the person offering a toast said, "I notice that some people's glasses are empty. That is not allowed!"
- At a banquet, several bottles of wine were provided free of charge

on every table, but those who wanted an alcohol-free beverage had to purchase it from a cash bar.

- An e-mail was sent to all faculty, encouraging them to attend an academic senate meeting, offering free beer as an incentive.

Don found that he dealt best with these situations by consciously changing his reactions to them. Rather than feeling pressured to drink because of these social messages, he decided to view them as cultural practices that contribute to the scope of alcohol problems, no matter how benign they may seem. He came up with the following parallel: Just as rejecting once-innocent-sounding racist and sexist comments has become a social norm that has had an overall positive effect on our society, he could begin to think about ways to raise his colleagues' consciousness about the unintended effect of these practices. Don knew what he was talking about: his decision to abstain had come about in part because his faculty position had been in jeopardy due to several instances of his coming to work under the influence.

Personal Freedom or Invisible Prison?

Some people want to keep drinking just to show that they can. Abstaining from alcohol can take on extra meaning that is unpleasant. Sobriety may, in the drinker's mind, be equated with:

- A feeling of being restricted and deprived
- A sense of failure, or admitting to being "alcoholic"
- The claustrophobia of "I can *never* . . . "
- Having to grow up
- Saying good-bye to all fun and enjoyment

Such thoughts can create a sense of mental imprisonment, and people naturally rebel against a perceived restriction of their freedom. Sometimes, too, it's an obstacle if other people *want* you to abstain. There may be a sense of "I'll be damned if I'm going to do that just because they want me to," even if part of you knows it's the right thing to do.

All of these are the result of *thinking* about drinking and abstinence in a particular way. If drinking is equated with your personal worth, freedom, youth, success, or happiness, then of course you wouldn't want to give it up.

But people can choose to quit simply because they decide that their lives will just be better without alcohol. They come to the realization that they will have not less, but *more* freedom of choice if they let go of alcohol. Within 12-step programs, this is expressed as the realization "that our lives had become unmanageable" and that abstinence is a door to freedom.

It is no coincidence that the more severe form of alcohol disorder is called alcohol *dependence*. The person's life comes to be ever more centered on drinking, until alcohol seems to be essential to life. The alcohol-dependent person literally depends on alcohol—to feel normal, to escape, to cope, to get to sleep, to have fun, to live. What once seemed like freedom becomes enslaving. Of course, abstaining in the interest of personal freedom isn't always so dramatic.

> Chris explained her decision this way: "It was just easier to quit; it was too much work trying to maintain moderation. Abstaining freed me from having to make the constant choice to drink or not to drink, how much to drink, remembering how long since I had had the last drink, and so on. Abstinence was a choice for me, even if initially a reluctant one. For me, not drinking is how I control my drinking."

If you are to choose abstinence, what is important first and foremost is to build an alcohol-free lifestyle that is so rewarding that it is just too good to give up. People who are sober but not enjoying life are bound to think about the pleasure (real or imagined) of drinking. The more your life was centered around drinking, the longer it may take to make this adjustment. For those who may have been drinking heavily ever since their teenage years, abstinence may require them to discover a whole new way of living an adult's life. Given that they have never experienced adult life without using alcohol, this can be daunting.

A helpful thought is "If over half of adults don't drink, it is obviously possible to get through life without alcohol." Life is brimming with potential pleasures, meaning, relationships, and happiness that do not require the use of alcohol. Finding and embracing them is an important part of establishing an alcohol-free lifestyle. Only you can decide whether you are ready, willing, and able to do this. If you think you're ready and willing but not so sure you're able, turn to the next chapter for sources of help.

If You Have Decided to Abstain from Alcohol

First, recognize that the decision-making process can be very draining. We hope that having made your decision will provide you with a sense of

Personal Reflection

If you're mulling over the pros and cons of abstaining, you might consider the monetary expense versus savings. If I drank only the recommended maximum of two drinks a day for men and my wife the recommended maximum of 1 drink a day for women, in a year we would have nearly eleven hundred drinks (365 days × 3 drinks per day = 1,095 drinks). Assuming drinks can cost between $1 and $5 per drink, we would have spent $1,095 to $5,475 a year on alcohol. Over a 50-year period, then, we would have spent between $54,000 and $273,000 on alcohol, enough to buy two to ten cars, numerous fine vacations, or putting one or two kids through college.

—RFM

relief. But, of course, once you have made your decision, you need to find the means to make it work. There are several things to consider.

If you have been able to reduce your drinking significantly by using the earlier parts of this book, it should be easier to continue reducing it to zero. In other words, if you have been able to go down to one or two drinks per day, then it may be possible for you to "cut down" to no drinks per day with minimal discomfort. If you're not sure how easy it will be to abstain, you might dispose of all alcohol in your home (if you are the only one who drinks) or make arrangements with your family members or roommates for the alcohol to be put out of your sight. Even though the goal is ultimately to be able to abstain even when exposed to alcohol and when around others who are drinking, it can help at first to remove or greatly reduce your exposure to alcohol.

If you are still drinking significant amounts daily, it may be wise to ask for help from an alcohol treatment professional. Effective science-based treatment methods are available to help people quit drinking.[25] In addition, if you're still drinking heavily, it is important to ensure that you have the medical help you need if you encounter significant withdrawal symptoms. Chapter 30 offers guidelines for finding competent professional help.

In either case, we want to point out that the material in Part IV may be helpful in shifting to an alcohol-free lifestyle. Those chapters are intended to provide alternatives to alcohol and to reduce the need to drink excessively. The same set of abilities (to change yourself, to maintain a healthy level of pleasant activities, to sleep well, to relax, to manage anxiety and depression, and so on) can therefore be useful whether your goal is moderation or abstinence. After all, the idea is that you can do these things without needing to use alcohol.

Finally, we want to remind you that giving up any habit can be challenging, but it is not impossible. Many people stop drinking on their own. You are most likely to be able to do this if you:

- Have already cut down substantially
- Have friends or relatives who can provide support and encouragement
- Have personal resources you can call on to help you through the process, such as personal practices that can provide a sense of balance, whether a physical exercise routine, spiritual practices, community service commitments, hobbies, other recreational pursuits, or something similar
- Have a fairly stable lifestyle, including a steady job schedule, regular contacts with other people, and goals toward which you are working
- Have a history of being able to give up habits such as smoking or other drugs on your own

If these descriptions do not fit you, it may be more challenging to stop drinking on your own, and we recommend that you obtain professional consultation or join a mutual support group focused on abstinence; see Chapter 30.

We wish you the best in your efforts to shift to an alcohol-free lifestyle. Making this decision as a rational personal choice is far preferable to waiting for some major negative life event to happen and therefore being forced to do so. It may even prevent such an event from occurring.

30

•

Sources of Help

Every year more than a million Americans seek some kind of help in getting and staying sober. Most of them have tried to change on their own without lasting success; thus they do the sensible thing and go in search of help and support to make the changes they desire.

The good news is that effective treatment is available. Whereas 50 years ago there were no science-based treatment methods for alcohol problems, today there is a menu of well-supported methods to choose from. Some, such as the self-control method described in this book, are designed to help people moderate their drinking. Others are available to help people abstain from alcohol.[26] In this chapter we describe briefly some of the options to explore, treatment methods with the strongest scientific evidence that they are helpful and not harmful.

The less-good news is that there is still a large gap between science-based effective methods and what is practiced in many community settings. That is, the alcohol treatment field has not caught up with the scientific advances made in recent decades. Thus many professionals and programs continue to deliver treatment methods with little evidence of effectiveness. This chapter is meant to help you find sources of effective treatment and support.

The 12-Step Program

The most familiar form of help for alcohol problems, at least in the United States, is Alcoholics Anonymous (AA) and its 12-step program for recovery. Founded in 1935, AA is not itself a treatment method but rather a fellowship of people supporting each other in recovery from alcohol dependence. AA groups are not run by treatment professionals but are peer-led by people who are themselves recovering from alcoholism. They follow 12 recommended steps that constitute a program for sober living, with strong emphasis on spirituality. Extensive information about the program is available at the AA website: *www.alcoholics-anonymous.org*. AA groups are available throughout the United States, with local phone help lines usually operating 24 hours a day. Groups are open and free to all who desire to quit drinking.

Many treatment programs also offer various forms of 12-step treatment that in some way incorporate the principles of AA. In the largest clinical trial ever conducted with treatments for alcohol dependence, 12-step facilitation therapy yielded the highest rate of abstinence among the three state-of-the-art methods tested.[27] The group as a whole maintained abstinence on 9 days out of 10, and about 40% abstained completely during the year after treatment. Research also rather consistently shows that people who attend and actively participate in AA meetings are more likely to remain abstinent, relative to those who do not attend AA. Thus there are very good reasons to explore AA and its 12-step program as an approach to recovery.

Some are put off, however, by the "God language" of AA. Although AA is not a religion, and not affiliated with any religious group, spirituality is clearly central to the 12-step approach, which is fairly described as a program not just for abstinence but for living. The 12 steps refer openly to God or a "Higher Power" with whom members seek to establish a closer relationship. AA is sensitive to this issue and openly welcomes atheists, agnostics, and people with any or no religious background. Indeed, although atheists and agnostics are less likely to attend AA, those who do have been found to benefit just as much as others.[28] They manage in part because AA is extremely permissive regarding how members think about their "Higher Power."

Based on the evidence, we encourage anyone who wants to quit drinking to give AA a try. We also believe that no one should be required to do so.

The Community Reinforcement Approach

A well-tested treatment method for helping people with alcohol problems is known as the community reinforcement approach (CRA).[29] First developed in the 1960s, CRA has a relatively simple philosophy: If you're going to give up something that you enjoy (in this case, drinking), it needs to be for a life that is even more enjoyable. That is, life without alcohol should be more fun and more rewarding than drinking was. The chapters in Part IV of this book speak directly to this issue. A dozen clinical trials have found CRA more effective than other treatment methods with which it has been compared in helping people to overcome alcohol and other drug dependence.

Although the philosophy sounds simple, CRA is actually a complex treatment method for which treatment professionals need special training.[30] A CRA counselor would help you build a life full of positive reinforcement that does not depend on drinking. This can involve learning some new coping skills, trying out old or new activities, or finding and keeping work that you enjoy. CRA goes far beyond helping you stop drinking. Its focus is on changing your life, social relationships, and environment in ways that make sobriety better than drinking. Ideally, you would develop a life without alcohol that is simply too good to give up. There is also a well-researched version of CRA for family members to help their loved one get sober.[31]

Learning Coping Skills

A closely related approach with a strong track record involves learning new skills for living a happy life without alcohol and to avoid returning to drinking. This is often called "cognitive-behavioral therapy," and is sometimes called "relapse prevention" treatment, although that name is used to describe many different approaches. The life skills that would be most helpful to you depend very much on your particular situation. There is no standard set of skills for everyone.

Some of the skills that are often helpful to people in establishing a sober lifestyle mirror those covered in Part IV of this book. Social skill training focuses on how to establish and maintain rewarding relationships. Couples can benefit from learning skills for communicating and living in intimate relationship. Other common components include skills for stress and mood management, assertiveness, and anger management. The overall point is to learn whatever skills you need to live an alcohol-free life.

Motivational Interviewing

Another common challenge is finding and maintaining the motivation to change your drinking. Often this has to do with working through ambivalence about drinking—you want to, and you don't want to. It's easy to get stuck in ambivalence.

Motivational interviewing[32] (MI) is a treatment approach introduced in 1983 precisely to help people resolve their ambivalence and move ahead with changes that they need to make in their lives. MI does not instill or provide motivation but rather is meant to help you find within yourself your own good reasons for change. Other people can give you reasons, but the ones that really count are the ones that matter to you—your own goals and values. MI is a relatively brief counseling approach, usually one to four sessions. MI can also be combined with other approaches, such as the community reinforcement approach and the learning of new life coping skills.

Medications

There are various medications to help people who want to quit drinking. The oldest and least expensive of these is disulfiram (trade name Antabuse). It works in a very simple way. You take it once a day, and if you don't drink, nothing happens. If you do drink, however, you become ill—headache, dizziness, nausea, and vomiting are common. In essence, disulfiram is an insurance policy. You make your decision (not to drink) once a day instead of many times a day. When taken regularly, enough of the drug stays in your system for a week or so to serve as a deterrent to impulsive drinking. It works, of course, only if you take the medication.

More recently there has been strong research support for naltrexone (trade name ReVia), which blocks opiate receptors in the brain. It seems to undermine alcohol's rewarding effects and to decrease urges to drink. A person who drinks while taking naltrexone doesn't become ill but typically just finds that alcohol is less enjoyable. Studies show that naltrexone can help people who are trying to get free from alcohol.[33] People who take it often describe decreased desire to drink, and if they do have a drink, they feel less inclined to drink heavily.

Most people who take one of these medications experience few or no side effects, and those that occur tend to be mild and short-lived. These medications are typically taken for a limited time, to help the person get through the challenging early months of abstinence, and it is generally recommended that they be taken in combination with other treatment, such as described previously. Naltrexone can be an expensive medication and is not always covered by insurance plans. If you are interested in the possibility of a medication to help you quit drinking, consult with your doctor, who would determine whether it is safe for you and could prescribe appropriate treatment.

Other Kinds of Help

Many other kinds of treatment and self-help are offered for people with alcohol problems. For example, the table below lists various kinds of mutual-help groups that are available in some areas. Although sampling these options can be easy enough, very little is known about their effectiveness, except for Alcoholics Anonymous, as described previously.

GETTING HELP

Mutual-help groups	Groups are led by ...	Groups are intended for ...	General approach	Emphasis on total abstinence
Alcoholics Anonymous	Peers	Anyone with a sincere desire to stop drinking	Spiritual, 12-step disease model	High
Calix Society	Professional affiliate	Catholics already in recovery	Catholic faith and 12 steps	High
Moderation Management	Professional moderator	People who want to reduce their drinking	Behavioral self-control	Low
Overcomers Outreach	Peers	Christians seeking to overcome an addiction	Christian faith and 12 steps	High
Rational Recovery	Professional affiliate	Anyone with an alcohol or other drug problem	Rational-emotive therapy	High
Secular Organizations for Sobriety	Peers	Anyone sincerely seeking sobriety	Secular approach to recovery	High

Mutual-help groups	Groups are led by . . .	Groups are intended for . . .	General approach	Emphasis on total abstinence
SMART Recovery	Trained coordinator	Anyone wanting to change addictive behavior	Rational-emotive behavior therapy	High
Women for Sobriety	Professional moderator	Women who desire to stop drinking	Empowerment, cognitive therapy	High

Source: Adapted from Miller, W. R. (Ed.). (2004). *Combined behavioral intervention: A clinical research guide for therapists treating individuals with alcohol abuse and dependence* (COMBINE Monograph Series, Vol. 1). Bethesda, MD: National Institute on Alcohol Abuse and Alcoholism.

Similarly, many kinds of treatment are offered for which there is little evidence of effectiveness. Particular caution is warranted with treatment methods that have been extensively evaluated and found ineffective. These include confrontational counseling, educational lectures and films, and psychodynamic (insight-oriented) psychotherapy. The most common problem, however, is that treatments are poorly defined and so difficult to evaluate. "Group psychotherapy," for example, is very common and can consist of almost anything. "Let the buyer beware" is good advice. It is still a relatively new idea that addiction treatment professionals or programs should deliver evidence-based services! Instead, "treatment" can and does consist of whatever the provider may believe in.

How, then, can you find your way through the jungle of options, to find treatment that is likely to help you? Here are some suggestions.

Ask Questions

It is perfectly legitimate and also wise to interview treatment providers about exactly what they do. Here are some questions you might ask.

- What is your approach to treating people with alcohol problems? (Here you are listening for clear, evidence-based treatment methods rather than vague descriptions. Ask for more than a brand name of treatment. What do they actually do?)
- To what extent is treatment the same for everyone, versus individualized? (In general, a one-size-fits-all program is undesirable.)

- How do you decide what treatment methods to use with a particular individual? (Although most providers say that they match treatments to the needs of the individual, what are the options available, and how is the decision made? To what extent do you have a say in the kind of treatment you receive?)
- What scientific evidence is there that the treatment methods you use are effective? (Don't settle for vague assurances or waffling about the limitations of scientific research. They should be able to specify what they do and point you to specific studies or reviews that support their approach.)
- What specific training have you had to provide this kind of treatment? (If they name a particular evidence-based treatment method, such as the CRA, MI, or coping skill training, find out how they learned it. Professionals don't acquire competence in methods such as these without specific training. Again, don't settle for vague assurances.)
- What will treatment cost? Will my health plan cover it?
- How long would you expect treatment to last? (Although there may not be an exact number of sessions or length of time, you should get clear information about at least average time for treatment.)

Ask Around

Another source of information is to ask about options from people who are likely to know professional reputations. You might ask a physician, pastor or rabbi, information center, or help line. Ask for recommendations through a local university that trains professionals in psychology, medicine, social work, or counseling. Within a health plan, you may need to start with your primary-care provider to get a referral. Ask specifically about professionals or programs that keep up on current research and provide science-based treatment. When you begin to hear the same names from several sources, check them out. There are also some excellent consumer information resources.[34]

Shop Around

Armed with options, it is reasonable to visit several professionals or programs. It is not necessary to stick with the first one you meet, any more than it is necessary to buy clothes at the first store you visit. In particular, it's important to have a good relationship with the person who is treating you. Consider:

- Do you feel respected and understood?
- Does he or she listen to your own perspectives and concerns?
- Do you feel confident that this person can help you? Does he or she seem competent?
- Do you understand the kind of treatment you will receive? How is confidentiality maintained?

Although it is not uncommon to be dealing with uncomfortable issues in treatment, you should feel trust and confidence in and respect from those who are treating you.

Treatment Settings

Treatment is offered in various settings. *Inpatient* programs involve admission to a hospital, where the person stays for a span of days or weeks. In *residential* programs you live and sleep in a special facility while receiving treatment, typically with a stay of several weeks or more. There are also short-term *detoxification* facilities to get people safely through the process of withdrawal. *Outpatient* programs provide treatment to people who come for specific sessions or visits, while living at home or in the community. Outpatient visits may occur once a week or more, or less frequently as treatment proceeds. There are also *intensive outpatient* programs that provide a substantial number of treatment sessions for a short period of time; for example, 4 hours a day, 3 days a week, over the course of 1 month.

Studies of treatment outcome show rather consistently that it is not the setting but the kind of treatment that matters. In general, inpatient and outpatient treatment programs have similar success rates, and outpatient treatment is usually far less expensive. Although an inpatient or residential stay can be helpful, and in some cases is medically necessary, it is rarely essential for long-term recovery. After discharge from an inpatient or residential program, you still have to deal with life in your community, and it is widely recognized that "aftercare" (outpatient treatment) is an essential follow-up to residential treatment.

The Bottom Line

The bottom line is to find the kind of help that works for you. If one approach isn't helping you, there are others available. Start with the evidence-based methods described previously and try different approaches until you find what works for you.

Don't give up too easily. It is very common to experience some setbacks along the way. Although the ideal in abstinence-focused treatment or mutual-help programs is for the person to quit drinking and never drink again, it is a minority who actually accomplish this goal on the first try, or even the second or third try. More common is to experience longer and longer spans of time without alcohol and periods of drinking that become shorter and more moderate.

You should, however, see good progress in treatment within 3 months or so. Specifically, your use of alcohol should be going down, if not stopping altogether. That's a bare minimum for effective treatment. You should also feel more comfortable and confident in living without alcohol. If that's not happening within about 3 months, try a different approach. Most drinkers who benefit from a particular treatment show substantial improvement within 2 to 3 months.

Finally, there's nothing unusual about going through several different kinds or episodes of treatment. The average smoker makes between eight and 11 serious attempts to quit before finally getting free of nicotine. It's very common to be treated several times.[35] This is, after all, a chronic condition. No one expects to be treated just once for diabetes, hypertension, or asthma and go away cured. As with those chronic diseases, the key is to stick with the things that help you stay healthy and sober.

APPENDIX A

•

The Wrath of Grapes:
Reasons for Concern

During the first three decades of the 20th century, public education regarding alcohol emphasized and sometimes exaggerated the dangers of ethyl alcohol. Alcohol was presented as a highly dangerous drug for anyone who used it. When national prohibition was repealed in 1933, however, alcohol education changed rapidly and soon became *alcoholism* education. In both public and professional views, a sharp distinction was drawn between "alcoholics" and other people. Alcohol came to be seen as dangerous only for certain individuals—those with alcoholism—and not for the rest of humanity.

In the late 20th and early 21st centuries, however, both public and professional views have swung back to acknowledging the serious dangers of alcohol as a drug. Alcohol consumption within the U.S. population has been declining steadily for decades. Per-capita consumption of alcohol is now less than half of what it was in the 1970s when we began this work, about 60% of all Americans now either abstain completely from alcohol or average less than one drink per week, and even regular drinkers are drinking far less (see the "How Many Adults Drink That Much or More?" table in Chapter 4).

There are good reasons for this caution. After tobacco, alcohol is the leading cause of preventable and premature death in America. Although very moderate drinkers (one to two standard drinks per day) show no higher health risks than abstainers, the rates of dependence, disease, disability, and premature death rise steadily from about three standard drinks per day upward. Clearly people are far better off abstaining than drinking heavily.

Health Problems Associated with Heavy Drinking

Alcohol is a highly effective solvent and a central nervous system depressant. Once consumed, it is distributed rapidly throughout the body. It goes wherever there is water in the body, which is nearly everywhere, and therefore is able to damage virtually all organ systems. Tolerance to alcohol (being able to "hold your liquor") does not decrease damage to the body. It merely allows the person to look and feel sober even when relatively high levels of alcohol are present in the body and doing their damage.

Central Nervous System

Some of the earliest damaging effects of alcohol are seen in the central nervous system. Alcohol affects the entire brain and is a "neurotoxin"—it destroys brain tissue. The higher and more frequent the dose of alcohol, the greater the damage. The magnitude of this damage became clear with methods for "imaging" the brain—seeing what is happening inside the brain without physically opening the skull. Brain images of people in treatment for alcohol dependence have shown substantial shrinkage of the brain. So many brain cells had been destroyed that the brain is physically smaller than it ought to be. Within the brain tissue that remains, the density of living nerve cells is also decreased. In short, by the time alcohol-dependent people get into treatment, their brains already tend to be smaller in size, with fewer nerve cell connections in what remains.

Well before such imaging was possible, there were clear indications that alcohol damages mental abilities. Declines in intelligence are less evident in verbal (language) skills than on nonverbal performance measures. That is, the harm that alcohol does to one's mental abilities may not be apparent in everyday conversation until the damage is rather far along. Affected much sooner are cognitive functions, including memory, concentration, abstract thinking, problem solving, orientation in three-dimensional space, speed, and dexterity in fine movements. On Intelligence Quotient (IQ) tests, these are known as "Performance IQ" measures, as distinct from "Verbal IQ." These effects can appear as difficulties in learning new material, in solving complex problems, or in concentrating and remembering things. Such effects may not be self-evident without careful testing, unless one's work happens to require some of the specific abilities that are affected early, such as rapid or carefully controlled finger movements, thinking in three dimensions, or solving problems that require a lot of concentration.

The effects of heavy drinking on the brain strongly resemble premature aging. The brain of a 40-year-old heavy drinker may resemble that of a normal 60-year-old. The good news is that cognitive functions damaged by alcohol do tend to improve with abstinence. There is now evidence that heavy drinkers who abstain from alcohol show significant enlargement of the brain, increasing density of nerve cell connections, and markedly improved mental

program of Alcoholics Anonymous predicts subsequent abstinence, and people who sustain recovery tend to show spiritual growth.

Alcohol and Mental Health

People with diagnosable alcohol use disorders also have higher rates of a wide range of other mental health problems. Anxiety and mood disorders are particularly common, but psychoses (like schizophrenia) and personality disorders also occur at elevated rates. About half of suicides occur with intoxication or are otherwise linked to alcohol/drug problems. Sleep disorders are common.

There is a "chicken and egg" question here. Do such mental health problems come first, with overdrinking following as a response to distress and an attempt to cope? Or does overdrinking cause or at least exacerbate other psychological problems? The answer seems to be "Yes" to both. Either can come first, and each will exacerbate and complicate treatment of the other. Fortunately, treating both will improve both as well.

Alcohol and Social Functioning

Finally, it is no surprise that overdrinking is associated with a host of social problems. A substantial proportion of all crimes, particularly violent crimes, are associated with alcohol use. Work functioning is often compromised, which can lead to job loss and unemployment. Financial problems are common. This takes a toll not only on the drinker but on loved ones as well. Family problems and domestic violence are greatly increased. Research indicates that family communication tends to be distressed and disturbed when an alcohol-dependent member is drinking, but relatively normal after he or she has been treated and sober.

These are some of the more common effects of prolonged heavy alcohol use. Alcohol affects virtually every system in the body, and beyond very moderate levels (one to two drinks per day) the effects are adverse. Heavy drinking compromises muscle tone and fitness and seems to accelerate aging. Pregnant women are advised to abstain completely from drinking during pregnancy because of unpredictable and potentially serious effects on the unborn child. Heavy drinkers are also at greatly increased risk for injury, disability, and death from a host of causes, including falls, burns, drowning, vehicle crashes, and pedestrian collisions. Overdrinking takes its toll not only on the drinker's mental health, but also on the health and welfare of his or her family.

APPENDIX B

●

An Inventory
of Alcohol-Related Problems

Here are a number of events that drinkers sometimes experience. Read each one carefully and circle the number of each experience that has <u>EVER</u> happened to you.

Has this <u>EVER</u> happened to you?

1. I have had a hangover or felt bad after drinking.
2. I have felt bad about myself because of my drinking.
3. I have missed days of work or school because of my drinking.
4. My family or friends have worried or complained about my drinking.
5. The quality of my work has suffered because of my drinking.
6. My ability to be a good parent has been harmed by my drinking.
7. After drinking, I have had trouble with sleeping, staying asleep, or nightmares.
8. I have driven a motor vehicle after having three or more drinks.
9. My drinking has caused me to use other drugs more.
10. I have been sick and vomited after drinking.
11. I have been unhappy because of my drinking.
12. Because of my drinking, I have not eaten properly.
13. I have failed to do what is expected of me because of my drinking.
14. I have felt guilty or ashamed because of my drinking.
15. While drinking, I have said or done embarrassing things.
16. When drinking, my personality has changed for the worse.
17. I have taken foolish risks when I have been drinking.
18. I have gotten into trouble because of drinking.
19. While drinking or using drugs, I have said harsh or cruel things to someone.
20. When drinking, I have done impulsive things that I regretted later.

21. I have gotten into a physical fight while drinking.
22. My physical health has been harmed by my drinking.
23. I have had money problems because of my drinking.
24. My marriage or love relationship has been harmed by my drinking.
25. I have smoked tobacco more when I am drinking.
26. My physical appearance has been harmed by my drinking.
27. My family has been hurt by my drinking.
28. A friendship or close relationship has been damaged by my drinking.
29. I have been overweight because of my drinking.
30. My sex life has suffered because of my drinking.
31. I have lost interest in activities and hobbies because of my drinking.
32. My spiritual or moral life has been harmed by my drinking.
33. Because of my drinking, I have not had the kind of life that I want.
34. My drinking has gotten in the way of my growth as a person.
35. My drinking has damaged my social life, popularity, or reputation.
36. I have spent too much or lost a lot of money because of my drinking.
37. I have been arrested for driving under the influence of alcohol.
38. I have had trouble with the law (other than driving while intoxicated) because of my drinking.
39. I have lost a marriage or a close love relationship because of my drinking.
40. I have been suspended or fired from or left a job or school because of my drinking.
41. I have lost a friend because of my drinking.
42. I have had an accident while drinking or intoxicated.
43. While drinking or intoxicated, I have been physically hurt, injured, or burned.
44. While drinking or intoxicated, I have injured someone else.
45. I have broken things while drinking or intoxicated.

Now count up the number of items you circled. That's your total score. People who are entering treatment for alcohol problems tend to score 20 or higher.

APPENDIX C

•

Tables for Estimating Blood Alcohol Concentration (BAC)

Instructions

Among the following tables, find the one that is for your own gender (women or men) and is closest to your body weight in pounds. (You can also obtain a personal table for your exact weight at *http://casaa.unm.edu/BACTable* by entering your gender and body weight and pressing "Create Table." All "drinks" in the table are standard drinks; see Chapter 4.)

To estimate your BAC level from a particular drinking occasion: Go down the left-hand column to find the total number of standard drinks you consumed. Then go across that row until you reach the column for the number of hours over which you consumed those drinks. The zero (0) hours column gives you the approximate BAC level if you consumed all the drinks at once.

Watch your BAC level go up: Pick a column for a certain period of drinking (such as 2 hours). As you go down that column you see the effect of adding one more standard drink during that period of time.

Watch your BAC level go down: Find your BAC level, then move across that row to the right. Each new column shows your approximate BAC level after one more hour has passed. (It subtracts 16 units per hour.)

To find the number of drinks that will keep you within your BAC limit: Find the column for the total number of hours of drinking. Go down that column and stop just before the BAC value goes over your limit. That row shows you the maximum number of drinks to stay within your limit during this period of time.

251

BAC Estimation Table for Women with a Body Weight of 100 lb (45 kilos)

	Number of hours										
	0	1	2	3	4	5	6	7	8	9	10
1 drink	45	29	13	0	0	0	0	0	0	0	0
2 drinks	90	74	58	42	26	10	0	0	0	0	0
3 drinks	135	119	103	87	71	55	39	23	7	0	0
4 drinks	180	164	148	132	116	100	84	68	52	36	20
5 drinks	225	209	193	177	161	145	129	113	97	81	65
6 drinks	270	254	238	222	206	190	174	158	142	126	110
7 drinks	315	299	283	267	251	235	219	203	187	171	155
8 drinks	360	344	328	312	296	280	264	248	232	216	200
9 drinks	405	389	373	357	341	325	309	293	277	261	245
10 drinks	450	434	418	402	386	370	354	338	322	306	290
11 drinks	495	479	463	447	431	415	399	383	367	351	335
12 drinks	540	524	508	492	476	460	444	428	412	396	380
13 drinks	585	569	553	537	521	505	489	473	457	441	425
14 drinks			598	582	566	550	534	518	502	486	470
15 drinks						595	579	563	547	531	515
16 drinks									592	576	560

BAC values over 600 mg% are not shown because they are normally fatal without very high alcohol tolerance.

BAC Estimation Table for Women with a Body Weight of 120 lb (54 kilos)

	Number of hours										
	0	1	2	3	4	5	6	7	8	9	10
1 drink	38	22	6	0	0	0	0	0	0	0	0
2 drinks	75	59	43	27	11	0	0	0	0	0	0
3 drinks	113	97	81	65	49	33	17	1	0	0	0
4 drinks	150	134	118	102	86	70	54	38	22	6	0
5 drinks	188	172	156	140	124	108	92	76	60	44	28
6 drinks	225	209	193	177	161	145	129	113	97	81	65
7 drinks	263	247	231	215	199	183	167	151	135	119	103
8 drinks	300	284	268	252	236	220	204	188	172	156	140
9 drinks	338	322	306	290	274	258	242	226	210	194	178
10 drinks	375	359	343	327	311	295	279	263	247	231	215
11 drinks	413	397	381	365	349	333	317	301	285	269	255
12 drinks	450	434	418	402	386	370	354	338	322	306	290
13 drinks	488	472	456	440	424	408	392	376	360	344	328
14 drinks	525	509	493	477	461	445	429	413	397	381	365
15 drinks	562	546	530	514	498	482	466	450	434	418	402
16 drinks	600	584	568	552	536	520	504	488	472	456	440
17 drinks				590	574	558	542	526	510	494	478
18 drinks						595	579	563	547	531	515
19 drinks									585	569	553
20 drinks											590

BAC values over 600 mg% are not shown because they are normally fatal without very high alcohol tolerance.

BAC Estimation Table for Women with a Body Weight of 140 lb (64 kilos)

	Number of hours										
	0	1	2	3	4	5	6	7	8	9	10
1 drink	32	16	0	0	0	0	0	0	0	0	0
2 drinks	64	48	32	16	0	0	0	0	0	0	0
3 drinks	96	80	64	48	32	16	0	0	0	0	0
4 drinks	129	113	97	81	65	49	33	17	1	0	0
5 drinks	161	145	129	113	97	81	65	49	33	17	1
6 drinks	193	177	161	145	129	113	97	81	65	49	33
7 drinks	225	209	193	177	161	145	129	113	97	81	65
8 drinks	257	241	225	209	193	177	161	145	129	113	97
9 drinks	289	273	257	241	225	209	193	177	161	145	129
10 drinks	321	305	289	273	257	241	225	209	193	177	161
11 drinks	354	338	322	306	290	274	258	242	226	210	194
12 drinks	386	370	354	338	322	306	290	274	258	242	226
13 drinks	418	402	386	370	354	338	322	306	290	274	258
14 drinks	450	434	418	402	386	370	354	338	322	306	290
15 drinks	482	466	450	434	418	402	386	370	354	338	322
16 drinks	514	498	482	466	450	434	418	402	386	370	354
17 drinks	546	530	514	498	482	466	450	434	418	402	386
18 drinks	579	563	547	531	515	499	483	467	451	435	419
19 drinks		595	579	563	547	531	515	499	483	467	451
20 drinks			595	579	563	547	531	515	499	483
21 drinks					595	579	563	547	531	515
22 drinks							595	579	563	547
23 drinks									595	579

BAC values over 600 mg% are not shown because they are normally fatal without very high alcohol tolerance.

BAC Estimation Table for Women with a Body Weight of 160 lb (73 kilos)

	Number of hours										
	0	1	2	3	4	5	6	7	8	9	10
1 drink	28	12	0	0	0	0	0	0	0	0	0
2 drinks	56	40	24	8	0	0	0	0	0	0	0
3 drinks	84	68	52	36	20	4	0	0	0	0	0
4 drinks	112	96	80	64	48	32	16	0	0	0	0
5 drinks	141	125	109	93	77	61	45	29	13	0	0
6 drinks	169	153	137	121	105	89	73	57	41	25	9
7 drinks	197	181	165	149	133	117	101	85	69	53	37
8 drinks	225	209	193	177	161	145	129	113	97	81	65
9 drinks	253	237	221	205	189	173	157	141	125	109	93
10 drinks	281	265	249	233	217	201	185	169	153	137	121
11 drinks	309	293	277	261	245	229	213	197	181	165	149
12 drinks	337	321	305	289	273	257	241	225	209	193	177
13 drinks	366	350	334	318	302	286	270	254	238	222	206
14 drinks	394	378	362	346	330	314	298	282	266	250	234
15 drinks	422	406	390	374	358	342	326	310	294	278	262
16 drinks	450	434	418	402	386	370	354	338	322	306	290
17 drinks	478	462	446	430	414	398	382	366	350	334	318
18 drinks	506	490	474	458	442	426	410	394	378	362	346
19 drinks	534	518	502	486	470	454	438	422	406	390	374
20 drinks	562	546	530	514	498	482	466	450	434	418	402
21 drinks	591	575	559	543	527	511	495	479	463	447	431
22 drinks			587	571	555	539	523	507	491	475	459
23 drinks			599	583	567	551	535	519	503	487
24 drinks					595	579	563	547	531	515
25 drinks							591	575	559	543

BAC values over 600 mg% are not shown because they are normally fatal without very high alcohol tolerance.

BAC Estimation Table for Women with a Body Weight of 180 lb (82 kilos)

	Number of hours										
	0	1	2	3	4	5	6	7	8	9	10
1 drink	25	9	0	0	0	0	0	0	0	0	0
2 drinks	50	34	18	2	0	0	0	0	0	0	0
3 drinks	75	59	43	27	11	0	0	0	0	0	0
4 drinks	100	84	68	52	36	20	4	0	0	0	0
5 drinks	125	109	93	77	61	45	29	13	0	0	0
6 drinks	150	134	118	102	86	70	54	38	22	6	0
7 drinks	175	159	143	127	111	95	79	63	47	31	15
8 drinks	200	184	168	152	136	120	104	88	72	56	40
9 drinks	225	209	193	177	161	145	129	113	97	81	65
10 drinks	250	234	218	202	186	170	154	138	122	106	90
11 drinks	275	259	243	227	211	195	179	163	147	131	115
12 drinks	300	284	268	252	236	220	204	188	172	156	140
13 drinks	325	309	293	277	261	245	229	213	197	181	165
14 drinks	350	334	318	302	286	270	254	238	222	206	190
15 drinks	375	359	343	327	311	295	279	263	247	331	215
16 drinks	400	384	368	352	336	320	304	288	272	256	240
17 drinks	425	409	393	377	361	345	329	313	297	281	265
18 drinks	450	434	418	402	386	370	354	338	322	306	290
19 drinks	475	459	443	427	411	395	379	363	347	331	315
20 drinks	500	484	468	452	436	420	404	388	372	356	340
21 drinks	525	509	493	477	461	445	429	413	397	381	365
22 drinks	550	534	518	502	486	470	454	438	422	406	390
23 drinks	575	559	543	527	511	495	479	463	447	431	415
24 drinks	600	585	568	552	536	520	504	488	472	456	440
25 drinks			593	577	561	545	529	513	497	481	465

BAC values over 600 mg% are not shown because they are normally fatal without very high alcohol tolerance.

BAC Estimation Table for Women with a Body Weight of 200 lb (91 kilos)

	Number of hours										
	0	1	2	3	4	5	6	7	8	9	10
1 drink	22	6	0	0	0	0	0	0	0	0	0
2 drinks	45	29	13	0	0	0	0	0	0	0	0
3 drinks	68	52	36	20	4	0	0	0	0	0	0
4 drinks	90	74	58	42	26	10	0	0	0	0	0
5 drinks	113	97	81	65	49	33	17	1	0	0	0
6 drinks	135	119	103	87	71	55	39	23	7	0	0
7 drinks	158	142	126	110	94	78	62	46	30	14	0
8 drinks	180	164	148	132	116	100	84	68	52	36	20
9 drinks	203	187	171	155	139	123	107	91	75	59	43
10 drinks	225	209	193	177	161	145	129	113	97	81	65
11 drinks	248	232	216	200	184	168	152	136	120	104	88
12 drinks	270	254	238	222	206	190	174	158	142	126	110
13 drinks	293	277	261	245	229	213	197	181	165	149	133
14 drinks	315	299	283	267	251	235	219	203	187	171	155
15 drinks	338	322	306	290	274	258	242	226	210	194	178
16 drinks	360	344	328	312	296	280	264	248	232	216	200
17 drinks	383	367	351	335	319	303	287	271	255	239	223
18 drinks	405	389	373	357	341	325	309	293	277	261	245
19 drinks	428	412	396	380	364	348	332	316	300	284	268
20 drinks	450	434	418	402	386	370	354	338	322	306	290
21 drinks	473	457	441	425	409	393	377	361	345	329	313
22 drinks	495	479	463	447	431	415	399	383	367	351	335
23 drinks	518	502	486	470	454	438	422	406	390	374	358
24 drinks	540	524	508	492	476	460	444	428	412	396	380
25 drinks	562	546	530	514	498	482	466	450	434	418	402

BAC Estimation Table for Women with a Body Weight of 220 lb (100 kilos)

	Number of hours										
	0	1	2	3	4	5	6	7	8	9	10
1 drink	20	4	0	0	0	0	0	0	0	0	0
2 drinks	41	25	9	0	0	0	0	0	0	0	0
3 drinks	61	45	29	13	0	0	0	0	0	0	0
4 drinks	82	66	50	34	18	2	0	0	0	0	0
5 drinks	102	86	70	54	38	22	6	0	0	0	0
6 drinks	123	107	91	75	59	43	27	11	0	0	0
7 drinks	143	127	111	95	79	63	47	31	15	0	0
8 drinks	164	148	132	116	100	84	68	52	36	20	4
9 drinks	184	168	152	136	120	104	88	72	56	40	24
10 drinks	205	189	173	157	141	125	109	93	77	61	45
11 drinks	225	209	193	177	161	145	129	113	97	81	65
12 drinks	245	229	213	197	181	165	149	133	117	101	85
13 drinks	266	250	234	218	202	186	170	154	138	122	106
14 drinks	286	270	254	238	222	206	190	174	158	142	126
15 drinks	307	291	275	259	243	227	211	195	179	163	147
16 drinks	327	311	295	279	263	247	231	215	199	183	167
17 drinks	348	332	316	300	284	268	252	236	220	204	188
18 drinks	368	352	336	320	304	288	272	256	240	224	208
19 drinks	389	373	357	341	325	309	293	277	261	245	229
20 drinks	409	293	377	361	345	329	313	297	281	265	249
21 drinks	430	414	398	382	366	350	334	318	302	286	270
22 drinks	450	434	418	402	386	370	354	338	322	306	290
23 drinks	470	454	438	422	406	390	374	358	342	326	310
24 drinks	491	475	459	443	427	411	395	379	363	347	331
25 drinks	511	495	479	463	447	431	415	399	383	367	351

BAC Estimation Table for Women with a Body Weight of 240 lb (109 kilos)

	Number of hours										
	0	1	2	3	4	5	6	7	8	9	10
1 drink	19	3	0	0	0	0	0	0	0	0	0
2 drinks	38	22	6	0	0	0	0	0	0	0	0
3 drinks	56	40	24	8	0	0	0	0	0	0	0
4 drinks	75	59	43	27	11	0	0	0	0	0	0
5 drinks	94	78	62	46	30	14	0	0	0	0	0
6 drinks	113	97	81	65	49	33	17	1	0	0	0
7 drinks	131	115	99	83	67	51	35	19	3	0	0
8 drinks	150	134	118	102	86	70	54	38	22	6	0
9 drinks	169	153	137	121	105	89	73	57	41	25	9
10 drinks	188	172	156	140	124	108	92	76	60	44	28
11 drinks	206	190	174	158	142	126	110	94	78	62	46
12 drinks	225	209	193	177	161	145	129	113	97	81	65
13 drinks	244	228	212	196	180	164	148	132	116	100	84
14 drinks	263	247	231	215	199	183	167	151	135	119	103
15 drinks	281	265	249	233	217	201	185	169	153	137	121
16 drinks	300	284	268	252	236	220	204	188	172	156	140
17 drinks	319	303	287	271	255	239	223	207	191	175	156
18 drinks	338	322	306	290	274	258	242	226	210	194	178
19 drinks	356	340	324	308	292	276	260	244	228	212	196
20 drinks	375	359	343	327	311	295	279	263	247	231	215
21 drinks	394	378	362	346	330	314	298	282	266	250	234
22 drinks	413	397	381	365	349	333	317	301	285	269	253
23 drinks	431	415	399	383	367	351	335	319	303	287	271
24 drinks	450	434	418	402	386	370	354	338	322	306	290
25 drinks	469	453	437	421	405	389	373	357	341	325	309

BAC Estimation Table for Men with a Body Weight of 100 lb (45 kilos)

	Number of hours										
	0	1	2	3	4	5	6	7	8	9	10
1 drink	38	22	6	0	0	0	0	0	0	0	0
2 drinks	75	59	43	27	11	0	0	0	0	0	0
3 drinks	113	97	81	65	49	33	17	1	0	0	0
4 drinks	150	134	118	102	86	70	54	38	22	6	0
5 drinks	188	172	156	140	124	108	92	76	60	44	28
6 drinks	225	209	193	177	161	145	129	113	97	81	65
7 drinks	263	247	231	215	199	183	167	151	135	119	103
8 drinks	300	284	268	252	236	220	204	188	172	156	140
9 drinks	338	322	306	290	274	258	242	226	210	194	178
10 drinks	375	359	343	327	311	295	279	263	247	231	215
11 drinks	413	397	381	365	349	333	317	301	285	269	253
12 drinks	450	434	418	402	386	370	354	338	322	306	290
13 drinks	488	472	456	440	424	408	392	376	360	344	328
14 drinks	525	509	493	477	461	445	429	413	397	381	365
15 drinks	562	546	530	514	498	482	466	450	434	418	402
16 drinks	600	584	568	552	536	520	504	488	472	456	440
17 drinks				590	574	558	542	526	510	494	478
18 drinks						595	579	563	547	531	515
19 drinks									585	569	553
20 drinks											590

BAC values over 600 mg% are not shown because they are normally fatal without very high alcohol tolerance.

BAC Estimation Table for Men with a Body Weight of 120 lb (54 kilos)

	Number of hours										
	0	1	2	3	4	5	6	7	8	9	10
1 drink	31	15	0	0	0	0	0	0	0	0	0
2 drinks	62	46	30	14	0	0	0	0	0	0	0
3 drinks	94	78	62	46	30	14	0	0	0	0	0
4 drinks	125	109	93	77	61	45	29	13	0	0	0
5 drinks	156	140	124	108	92	76	60	44	28	12	0
6 drinks	188	172	156	140	124	108	92	76	60	44	28
7 drinks	219	203	187	171	155	139	123	107	91	75	59
8 drinks	250	234	218	202	186	170	154	138	122	106	90
9 drinks	281	265	249	233	217	201	185	169	153	137	121
10 drinks	312	296	280	264	248	232	216	200	184	168	152
11 drinks	344	328	312	296	280	264	248	232	216	200	184
12 drinks	375	359	343	327	311	295	279	263	247	231	215
13 drinks	406	390	374	358	342	326	310	294	278	262	246
14 drinks	438	422	406	390	374	358	342	326	310	294	278
15 drinks	469	453	437	421	405	389	373	357	341	325	309
16 drinks	500	484	468	452	436	420	404	388	372	356	340
17 drinks	531	515	499	483	467	451	435	419	403	387	371
18 drinks	562	546	530	514	498	482	466	450	434	418	402
19 drinks	594	578	562	546	530	514	498	482	466	450	434
20 drinks			593	577	561	545	529	513	497	481	465
21 drinks					592	576	560	544	528	512	496
22 drinks							592	576	560	544	528
23 drinks									591	575	559
24 drinks											590

BAC values over 600 mg% are not shown because they are normally fatal without very high alcohol tolerance.

BAC Estimation Table for Men with a Body Weight of 140 lb (64 kilos)

	Number of hours										
	0	1	2	3	4	5	6	7	8	9	10
1 drink	27	11	0	0	0	0	0	0	0	0	0
2 drinks	54	38	22	6	0	0	0	0	0	0	0
3 drinks	80	64	48	32	16	0	0	0	0	0	0
4 drinks	107	91	75	59	43	27	11	0	0	0	0
5 drinks	134	118	102	86	70	54	38	22	6	0	0
6 drinks	161	145	129	113	97	81	65	49	33	17	1
7 drinks	188	172	156	140	124	108	92	76	60	44	28
8 drinks	214	198	182	166	150	134	118	102	86	70	54
9 drinks	241	225	209	193	177	161	145	129	113	97	81
10 drinks	268	252	236	220	204	188	172	156	140	124	108
11 drinks	295	279	263	247	231	215	199	183	167	151	135
12 drinks	321	305	289	273	257	241	225	209	193	172	161
13 drinks	348	332	316	300	284	268	252	236	220	204	188
14 drinks	375	359	343	327	311	295	279	263	247	231	215
15 drinks	402	386	370	354	338	322	306	290	274	258	242
16 drinks	429	413	397	381	365	349	333	317	301	285	269
17 drinks	455	439	423	407	391	375	359	343	327	311	295
18 drinks	482	466	450	434	418	402	386	370	354	338	322
19 drinks	509	493	477	461	445	429	413	397	381	365	349
20 drinks	536	520	504	488	472	456	440	424	408	392	376
21 drinks	562	546	530	514	498	482	466	450	434	418	402
22 drinks	589	573	557	541	525	509	493	477	461	445	429
23 drinks		600	584	568	552	536	520	504	488	472	456
24 drinks			595	579	563	547	531	515	499	483
25 drinks					590	574	558	542	526	510

BAC values over 600 mg% are not shown because they are normally fatal without very high alcohol tolerance.

BAC Estimation Table for Men with a Body Weight of 160 lb (73 kilos)

	Number of hours										
	0	1	2	3	4	5	6	7	8	9	10
1 drink	23	7	0	0	0	0	0	0	0	0	0
2 drinks	47	31	15	0	0	0	0	0	0	0	0
3 drinks	70	54	38	22	6	0	0	0	0	0	0
4 drinks	94	78	62	46	30	14	0	0	0	0	0
5 drinks	117	101	85	69	53	37	21	5	0	0	0
6 drinks	141	125	109	93	77	61	45	29	13	0	0
7 drinks	164	148	132	116	100	84	68	52	36	20	4
8 drinks	188	172	156	140	124	108	92	76	60	44	28
9 drinks	211	195	179	163	147	131	115	99	83	67	51
10 drinks	234	218	202	186	170	154	138	122	106	90	74
11 drinks	258	242	226	210	194	178	162	146	130	114	98
12 drinks	281	265	249	233	217	201	185	169	153	137	121
13 drinks	305	289	273	257	241	225	209	193	177	161	145
14 drinks	328	312	296	280	264	248	232	216	200	184	168
15 drinks	352	336	329	304	288	272	256	240	224	208	192
16 drinks	375	359	343	327	311	295	279	263	247	231	215
17 drinks	398	382	366	350	334	318	302	286	270	254	238
18 drinks	422	406	390	374	358	342	326	310	294	278	262
19 drinks	445	429	413	397	381	365	349	333	317	301	285
20 drinks	469	453	437	421	405	389	373	357	341	325	309
21 drinks	492	476	460	444	428	412	396	380	364	348	332
22 drinks	516	500	484	468	452	436	420	404	388	372	356
23 drinks	539	523	507	491	475	459	443	427	411	395	379
24 drinks	562	546	530	514	498	482	466	450	434	418	402
25 drinks	586	570	554	538	522	506	490	474	458	442	426

BAC Estimation Table for Men with a Body Weight of 180 lb (82 kilos)

	Number of hours										
	0	1	2	3	4	5	6	7	8	9	10
1 drink	21	5	0	0	0	0	0	0	0	0	0
2 drinks	42	26	10	0	0	0	0	0	0	0	0
3 drinks	62	46	30	14	0	0	0	0	0	0	0
4 drinks	83	67	51	35	19	3	0	0	0	0	0
5 drinks	104	88	72	56	40	24	8	0	0	0	0
6 drinks	125	109	93	77	61	45	29	13	0	0	0
7 drinks	146	130	114	98	82	66	50	34	18	2	0
8 drinks	167	151	135	119	103	87	71	55	39	23	7
9 drinks	188	172	156	140	124	108	92	76	60	44	28
10 drinks	208	192	176	160	144	128	112	96	80	64	48
11 drinks	229	213	197	181	165	149	133	117	101	85	69
12 drinks	250	234	218	202	186	170	154	138	122	106	90
13 drinks	271	255	239	223	207	191	175	159	143	127	111
14 drinks	292	276	260	244	228	212	196	180	164	148	132
15 drinks	312	296	280	264	248	232	216	200	184	168	152
16 drinks	333	317	301	285	269	253	237	221	205	189	173
17 drinks	354	338	322	306	290	274	258	242	226	210	194
18 drinks	375	359	343	327	311	295	279	263	247	231	215
19 drinks	396	380	364	348	332	316	300	284	268	252	236
20 drinks	417	401	385	369	353	337	321	305	289	273	257
21 drinks	438	422	406	390	374	358	342	326	310	294	278
22 drinks	458	442	426	410	394	378	362	346	330	314	298
23 drinks	479	463	447	431	415	399	383	367	351	335	319
24 drinks	500	484	468	452	436	420	404	388	372	356	340
25 drinks	521	505	489	473	457	441	425	409	393	377	361

BAC Estimation Table for Men with a Body Weight of 200 lb (91 kilos)

	Number of hours										
	0	1	2	3	4	5	6	7	8	9	10
1 drink	19	3	0	0	0	0	0	0	0	0	0
2 drinks	38	22	6	0	0	0	0	0	0	0	0
3 drinks	56	40	24	8	0	0	0	0	0	0	0
4 drinks	75	59	43	27	11	0	0	0	0	0	0
5 drinks	94	78	62	46	30	14	0	0	0	0	0
6 drinks	113	97	81	65	49	33	17	1	0	0	0
7 drinks	131	115	99	83	67	51	35	19	3	0	0
8 drinks	150	134	118	102	86	70	54	38	22	6	0
9 drinks	169	153	137	121	105	89	73	57	41	25	9
10 drinks	188	172	156	140	124	108	92	76	60	44	28
11 drinks	206	190	174	158	142	126	110	94	78	62	46
12 drinks	225	209	193	177	161	145	129	113	97	81	65
13 drinks	244	228	212	196	180	164	148	132	116	100	84
14 drinks	263	247	231	215	199	183	167	151	135	119	103
15 drinks	281	265	249	233	217	201	185	169	153	137	121
16 drinks	300	284	268	252	236	220	204	188	172	156	140
17 drinks	319	303	287	271	255	239	223	207	191	175	156
18 drinks	338	322	306	290	274	258	242	226	210	194	178
19 drinks	356	340	324	308	292	276	260	244	228	212	196
20 drinks	375	359	343	327	311	295	279	263	247	231	215
21 drinks	394	378	362	346	330	314	298	282	266	250	234
22 drinks	413	397	381	365	349	333	317	301	285	269	253
23 drinks	431	415	399	383	367	351	335	319	303	287	271
24 drinks	450	434	418	402	386	370	354	338	322	306	290
25 drinks	469	453	437	421	405	389	373	357	431	325	309

BAC Estimation Table for Men with a Body Weight of 220 lb (100 kilos)

	Number of hours										
	0	1	2	3	4	5	6	7	8	9	10
1 drink	17	1	0	0	0	0	0	0	0	0	0
2 drinks	34	18	2	0	0	0	0	0	0	0	0
3 drinks	51	35	19	3	0	0	0	0	0	0	0
4 drinks	68	52	36	20	4	0	0	0	0	0	0
5 drinks	85	69	53	37	21	5	0	0	0	0	0
6 drinks	102	86	70	54	38	22	6	0	0	0	0
7 drinks	119	103	87	71	55	39	23	7	0	0	0
8 drinks	136	120	104	88	72	56	40	24	8	0	0
9 drinks	153	137	121	105	89	73	57	41	25	9	0
10 drinks	170	154	138	122	106	90	74	58	42	26	10
11 drinks	188	172	156	140	124	108	92	76	60	44	28
12 drinks	205	189	173	157	141	125	109	93	77	61	45
13 drinks	222	206	190	174	158	142	126	110	94	78	62
14 drinks	239	223	207	191	175	159	143	127	111	95	79
15 drinks	256	240	224	208	192	176	160	144	128	112	96
16 drinks	273	257	241	225	209	193	177	161	145	129	113
17 drinks	290	274	258	242	226	210	194	178	162	146	130
18 drinks	307	291	275	259	243	227	211	195	179	163	147
19 drinks	324	308	292	276	260	244	228	212	196	180	164
20 drinks	341	325	309	293	277	261	245	229	213	197	181
21 drinks	358	342	326	310	294	278	262	246	230	214	198
22 drinks	375	359	343	327	311	295	279	263	247	231	215
23 drinks	392	376	360	344	328	312	296	280	264	248	232
24 drinks	409	393	377	361	345	329	313	297	281	265	249
25 drinks	426	410	394	378	362	346	330	314	298	282	266

BAC Estimation Table for Men with a Body Weight of 240 lb (109 kilos)

	Number of hours										
	0	1	2	3	4	5	6	7	8	9	10
1 drink	16	0	0	0	0	0	0	0	0	0	0
2 drinks	31	15	0	0	0	0	0	0	0	0	0
3 drinks	47	31	15	0	0	0	0	0	0	0	0
4 drinks	62	46	30	14	0	0	0	0	0	0	0
5 drinks	78	62	46	30	14	0	0	0	0	0	0
6 drinks	94	78	62	46	30	14	0	0	0	0	0
7 drinks	109	93	77	61	45	29	13	0	0	0	0
8 drinks	125	109	93	77	61	45	29	13	0	0	0
9 drinks	141	125	109	93	77	61	45	29	13	0	0
10 drinks	156	140	124	108	92	76	60	44	28	12	0
11 drinks	172	156	140	124	108	92	76	60	44	28	12
12 drinks	188	172	154	140	124	108	92	76	60	44	28
13 drinks	203	187	171	155	139	123	107	91	75	59	43
14 drinks	219	203	187	171	155	139	123	107	91	75	59
15 drinks	234	218	202	186	170	154	138	122	106	90	74
16 drinks	250	234	218	202	186	170	154	138	122	106	90
17 drinks	266	250	234	218	202	186	170	154	138	122	106
18 drinks	281	265	249	233	217	201	185	169	153	137	121
19 drinks	297	281	265	249	233	217	201	185	169	153	137
20 drinks	312	296	280	264	248	232	216	200	184	168	152
21 drinks	328	312	296	280	264	248	232	216	200	184	168
22 drinks	344	328	312	296	280	264	248	232	216	200	184
23 drinks	359	343	327	311	295	279	263	247	231	215	199
24 drinks	375	359	343	327	311	295	279	263	247	231	215
25 drinks	391	375	359	343	327	311	295	279	263	247	231

Going Further:
Recommended Resources

Alcohol Problems

Books

AA World Services. (2001). *Alcoholics Anonymous: The story of how many thousands of men and women have recovered from alcoholism* (4th ed.). New York: Author.

Fletcher, A. M. (2001). *Sober for good: New solutions for drinking problems—Advice from those who have succeeded.* Boston: Houghton/Harcourt.

Fletcher, A. M. (2013). *Inside rehab: The surprising truth about addiction treatment—and how to get the help that works.* New York: Viking Penguin.

Meyers, R. J., & Wolfe, B. L. (2004). *Get your loved one sober: Alternatives to nagging, pleading and threatening.* Center City, MN: Hazelden.

Prochaska, J. O., Norcross, J., & DiClemente, C. (1994). *Changing for good: A revolutionary six-stage program for overcoming bad habits and moving your life positively forward.* New York: Avon Books.

Rotgers, F., Kern, M. F., & Hoeltzel, R. (2002). *Responsible drinking: A moderation management approach for problem drinkers.* Oakland, CA: New Harbinger.

Sanchez-Craig, M. (1995). *Drink wise: How to quit drinking or cut down* (2nd ed.). Toronto: Centre for Addiction and Mental Health.

Volpicelli, J., & Szalavitz, M. (2000). *Recovery options: The complete guide.* New York: Wiley.

Websites

Alcoholics Anonymous
> *www.aa.org* (United States)
> *www.alcoholics-anonymous.org.uk* (Great Britain)
> *www.alcoholicsanonymous.ie* (Ireland)

www.aacanada.com (Canada)
www.aa.org.au (Australia)
http://aa.org.nz (New Zealand)

Alcohol Drug Association New Zealand
www.adanz.org.nz

Australian Centre for Addiction Research
www.acar.net.au

Canadian Centre on Substance Abuse
www.ccsa.ca

Drinker's Check-up
www.drinkerscheckup.com

Moderation Management
www.moderation.org

National Drug Advisory and Treatment Centre (Ireland)
www.addictionireland.ie

National Institutes of Health Website on Substance Abuse: authoritative information on addictions and types of substance abuse
http://health.nih.gov/category/SubstanceAbuse

National Treatment Agency for Substance Misuse (Great Britain)
www.nta.nhs.uk

Secular Organizations for Sobriety
www.cfiwest.org/sos/brochures/overview.htm

Smart Recovery
www.smartrecovery.org (United States)
http://smartrecoveryaustralia.com.au (Australia)
www.smartrecovery.ca (Alberta, Canada)
www.smartrecoveryontario.com (Ontario, Canada)
www.smartrecoveryquebec.org (Quebec, Canada)
www.smartrecovery.org.uk (Great Britain)

Women for Sobriety
www.womenforsobriety.org

Mental Health

Books

Abramowitz, J. S. (2012). *The stress less workbook: Simple strategies to relieve pressure, manage commitments, and minimize conflicts.* New York: Guilford Press.

Alberti, R. E., & Emmons, M. L. (2008). *Your perfect right: Assertiveness and equality in your life and relationships* (9th ed.). Atascadero, CA: Impact.

Benson, H., & Klipper, M. Z. (2000). *The relaxation response.* New York: Quill.

Bien, T. H., & Bien, B. (2003). *Finding the center within: The healing way of mindfulness meditation.* Hoboken, NJ: Wiley.

Burns, D. D. (2006). *When panic attacks: The new, drug-free anxiety therapy that can change your life.* New York: Morgan Road Books.

Burns, D. D. (1999). *Feeling good: The new mood therapy.* New York: Avon Books.

Clark, D. A., & Beck, A. T. (2011). *The anxiety and worry workbook: The cognitive-behavioral solution.* New York: Guilford Press.

Fanning, P., & McKay, M. (2008). Progressive relaxation and breathing (relaxation and stress reduction audio series). Oakland, CA: New Harbinger.

Gentry, D. (2007). *Anger management for dummies.* Indianapolis, IN: Wiley.

Germer, C. K. (2009). *The mindful path to self-compassion: Freeing yourself from destructive thoughts and emotions.* New York: Guilford Press.

Gottman, J. M., & Silver, N. (1999). *The seven principles for making marriage work: A practical guide from the country's foremost relationship expert.* New York: Three Rivers.

Greenberger, D., & Padesky, C. A. (1995). *Mind over mood: Change how you feel by changing the way you think.* New York: Guilford Press.

Ilardi, S. S. (2010). *The depression cure: The 6-step program to beat depression without drugs.* Cambridge: Da Capo Lifelong Books.

Jacobs, G. D. (1999). *Say good night to insomnia.* New York: Holt.

Kabat-Zinn, J. (2006). *Mindfulness for beginners* [audio book]. Louisville, CO: Sounds True.

Kurtz, E., & Ketcham, K. (1992). *The spirituality of imperfection: Storytelling and the journey to wholeness.* New York: Bantam Books.

Lewinsohn, P. M., Muñoz, R. F., Youngren, M. A., & Zeiss, A. M. (1992). *Control your depression* (rev. ed.). New York: Fireside.

Miller, W. R. (2008). *Living as if: Your road, your life* [client journal and facilitator guide]. Carson City, NV: The Change Companies.

Miller, W. R., & C'de Baca, J. (2001). *Quantum change: When epiphanies and sudden insights transform ordinary lives.* New York: Guilford Press.

Miller, W. R., & Mee-Lee, D. (2010). *Self-management: A guide to your feelings, motivation and positive mental health* [client journal and facilitator guide]. Carson City, NV: The Change Companies.

Nay, W. R. (2012). *Taking charge of anger: Six steps to asserting yourself without losing control* (2nd ed.). New York: Guilford Press.

Nichols, M. P. (2009). *The lost art of listening: How learning to listen can improve relationships* (2nd ed.). New York: Guilford Press.

Orsillo, S. M., & Roemer, L. (2011). *The mindful way through anxiety: Break free from chronic worry and reclaim your life.* New York: Guilford Press.

Siegel, R. D. (2010). *The mindfulness solution: Everyday practices for everyday problems.* New York: Guilford Press.

Williams, J. M. G., Teasdale, J. D., Segal, Z. V., & Kabat-Zinn, J. (2007). *The mindful way through depression: Freeing yourself from chronic unhappiness.* New York: Guilford Press.

Wright, J. H., & McCray, L. W. (2011). *Breaking free from depression: Pathways to wellness.* New York: Guilford Press.

Websites

UNITED STATES

Depression and Bipolar Support Alliance: dedicated to providing support to improve the lives of people who have mood disorders
www.dbsalliance.org

National Institutes of Health website on mental health and behavior: authoritative information on mental health issues, including a list of disorders and information about them
http://health.nih.gov/category/MentalHealthandBehavior

UNITED KINGDOM

Depression Alliance
www.depressionalliance.org

Depression UK
www.depressionuk.org

CANADA

Mood Disorders Society of Canada
www.mooddisorderscanada.ca

STOP-SMOKING SITES

Smokefree.gov: *http://smokefree.gov*
    Also in Spanish: *http://espanol.smokefree.gov*

Become an ex, from the Legacy Foundation: *www.becomeanex.org*
    Also in Spanish: *http://es.becomeanex.org*

Notes

1. National Institute on Alcohol Abuse and Alcoholism. (2005). *Helping patients who drink too much: A clinician's guide*. Bethesda, MD: National Institutes of Health.

2. Corrao, G., Bagnardi, V., Zambon, A., et al. (2004). A meta-analysis of alcohol consumption and the risk of 15 diseases. *Preventive Medicine, 38*, 613–619.

3. Miller, W. R., Walters, S. T., & Bennett, M. E. (2001). How effective is alcoholism treatment in the United States? *Journal of Studies on Alcohol, 62*, 211–220.

4. Miller, W. R., Leckman, A. L., Delaney, H. D., et al. (1992). Long-term follow-up of behavioral self-control training. *Journal of Studies on Alcohol, 53*, 249–261.

5. Fletcher, A. M. (2001). *Sober for good: New solutions for drinking problems—Advice from those who have succeeded*. Boston: Houghton/Harcourt.

6. Miller, W. R., Forcehimes, A. A., & Zweben, A. (2011). *Treating addiction: Guidelines for professionals*. New York: Guilford Press.

7. Miller, W. R., Walters, S. T., & Bennett, M. E. (2001). How effective is alcoholism treatment? *Journal of Studies on Alcohol, 62*, 211–220.

8. Selzer, M. L. (1971). The Michigan Alcoholism Screening Test: The quest for a new diagnostic instrument. *American Journal of Psychiatry, 127*(12), 1653–1658.

9. Horn, J. K., Skinner, H. A., Wanberg, K., et al. (1984). *The Alcohol Dependence Scale (ADS)*. Toronto: Centre for Addiction and Mental Health. Copyright 1984 by the Centre for Addiction and Mental Health and Harvey A. Skinner. Reprinted by permission.

10. Skinner, H. A., & Horn, J. K. (1984). *Alcohol Dependence Scale (ADS) user's guide*. Toronto: Addiction Research Foundation.

11. Even the authors of *Alcoholics Anonymous* left the door open for moderation by those who were not truly alcoholic: "If anyone who is showing inability to control his drinking can do the right-about-face and drink

like a gentleman, our hats are off to him" (Alcoholics Anonymous. [1939]. *Alcoholics Anonymous.* New York: AA World Services). Similarly, Marty Mann's advice was very pragmatic: If you think you can do it, give it a try (Mann, M. [1958]. *Marty Mann's new primer on alcoholism.* New York: Holt, Rinehart & Winston).

12. Sanchez-Craig, M. (1980). Random assignment to abstinence or controlled drinking in a cognitive-behavioral program: Short-term effects on drinking behavior. *Addictive Behaviors, 5,* 35–39.

13. Miller, W. R., Heather, N., & Hall, W. (1991). Calculating standard drink units: International comparisons. *British Journal of Addiction, 86,* 43–47.

14. Lansky, D., Nathan, P. E., & Lawson, D. M. (1978). Blood alcohol level discrimination by alcoholics: The role of internal and external cues. *Journal of Consulting and Clinical Psychology, 46,* 953–960.

15. Mann, R. E. (2002). Choosing a rational threshold for the definition of drunk driving: What research recommends. *Addiction, 97,* 1237–1238.

16. Miller, W. R. (1978). Behavioral treatment of problem drinkers: A comparative outcome study of three controlled drinking therapies. *Journal of Consulting and Clinical Psychology, 46,* 74–86.

17. Mark Twain in his book *Personal Recollections of Joan of Arc.*

18. Kivlahan, D. R., Marlatt, G. A., Fromme, K., et al. (1990). Secondary prevention with college drinkers: Evaluation of an alcohol skills training program. *Journal of Consulting and Clinical Psychology, 58,* 805–810.

19. Miller, W. R., & Pechacek, T. F. (1987). New roads: Assessing and treating psychological dependence. *Journal of Substance Abuse Treatment, 4,* 73–77.

20. Doyle, S. R., Donovan, D. M., & Simpson, T. L. (2011). Validation of a nine-dimensional measure of drinking motives for use in clinical applications: The Desired Effects of Drinking Scale. *Addictive Behaviors, 36*(11), 1052–1060.

21. Lewinsohn, P. M., Muñoz, R. F., Youngren, M. A., & Zeiss, A. M. (1992, rev. ed.). *Control your depression.* New York: Fireside Books.

    Cuijpers, P., Muñoz, R. F., Clarke, G., & Lewinsohn, P. M. (2009). Psychoeducational treatment and prevention of depression: The "Coping with Depression" course thirty years later. *Clinical Psychology Review, 29,* 449–458.

    Dimidjian, S., Barrera, M., Martell, C., Muñoz, R. F., & Lewinsohn, P. M. (2011). The origins and current status of behavioral activation treatments for depression. *Annual Review of Clinical Psychology, 7*(1), 1–38.

22. Kessler, R. C., Berglund, P., Demler, O., et al. (2003). The epidemiology of major depressive disorder: Results from the National Comorbidity Survey Replication (NCS-R). *Journal of the American Medical Association, 289*(23), 3095–3105.

23. Miller, W. R., & DiPilato, M. (1983). Treatment of nightmares via relaxation and desensitization: A controlled evaluation. *Journal of Consulting and Clinical Psychology, 51,* 870–877.

24. Mukamal, K. J., Congrave, K. M., Mittleman, M. A., et al. (2003). Roles of drinking pattern and type of alcohol consumed in coronary heart disease in men. *New England Journal of Medicine, 348*(2), 109–118.

25. Miller, W. R., Forcehimes, A. A., & Zweben, A. (2011). *Treating addiction: Guidelines for professionals.* New York: Guilford Press.

26. For example, Volpicelli, J., & Szalavitz, M. (2000). *Recovery options: The complete guide.* New York: Wiley.

27. Babor, T. F., & DelBoca, F. K. (Eds.). (2003). *Treatment matching in alcoholism.* Cambridge, UK: Cambridge University Press.

28. Tonigan, J. S., Miller, W. R., & Schermer, C. (2002). Atheists, agnostics, and Alcoholics Anonymous. *Journal of Studies on Alcohol, 63,* 534–541.

29. Meyers, R. J., & Miller, W. R. (Eds.). (2001). *A community reinforcement approach to addiction treatment.* Cambridge, UK: Cambridge University Press.

30. Meyers, R. J., & Smith, J. E. (1995). *Clinical guide to alcohol treatment: The community reinforcement approach.* New York: Guilford Press.

31. Meyers, R. J., & Wolfe, B. L. (2004). *Get your loved one sober: Alternatives to nagging, pleading and threatening.* Center City, MN: Hazelden.

32. Miller, W. R., & Rollnick, S. (2012). *Motivational interviewing: Helping people change* (3rd ed.). New York: Guilford Press.

33. Anton, R. F., O'Malley, S. S., Ciraulo, D. A., et al. (2006). Combined pharmacotherapies and behavioral interventions for alcohol dependence. The COMBINE study: A randomized controlled trial. *Journal of the American Medical Association, 295,* 2003–2017.

34. Fletcher, A. M. (2001). *Sober for good: New solutions for drinking problems—Advice from those who have succeeded.* Boston: Houghton/Harcourt.
    Fletcher, A. M. (2013). *Inside rehab: The surprising truth about addiction treatment and how to get help that works.* New York: Viking.

35. U.S. Department of Health and Human Services. (2001). *Women and smoking: A report of the Surgeon General.* Rockville, MD: U.S. Department of Health and Human Services, Public Health Service, Centers for Disease Control, Center for Chronic Disease Prevention and Health Promotion, Office on Smoking and Health. See *www.ncbi.nlm.nih.gov/books/NBK44303.*

Bibliography

Research on This Treatment Approach

The specific treatment approach described in this book, known technically as behavioral self-control training, has been tested in a large number of clinical trials, many with excellent documentation of treatment outcomes over followup periods of a year or more. Four decades after our first book on this topic, new clinical trials continue to appear apace. Here are references for clinical trials of moderation training, with both positive and negative findings.

Adams, D. R. (1990). *An early counseling intervention program for problem drinkers contrasting group and individual delivery formats (group treatment).* Unpublished doctoral dissertation, University of British Columbia, Canada.

Alden, L. (1978). Evaluation of a preventive self-management programme for problem drinkers. *Canadian Journal of Behavioural Science, 10,* 258–263.

Alden, L. (1980). Preventive strategies in the treatment of alcohol abuse: A review and a proposal. In P. Davidson & S. Davidson (Eds.), *Behavioral medicine: Changing health lifestyles* (pp. 256–278). New York: Brunner/Mazel.

Alden, L. E. (1988). Behavioral self-management controlled-drinking strategies in a context of secondary prevention. *Journal of Consulting and Clinical Psychology, 56,* 280–286.

Andreasson, S., Hansagi, H., & Osterlund, B. (2002). Short-term treatment for alcohol-related problems: Four-session guided self-change versus one session of advice—A randomized, controlled trial. *Alcoholism Treatment Quarterly, 28*(1), 57–62.

Baer, J. S., Kivlahan, D. R., Blume, A. W., et al. (2001). Brief intervention for heavy-drinking college students: 4-year follow-up and natural history. *American Journal of Public Health, 91,* 1310–1316.

Baker, T. B., Udin, H., & Vogler, R. E. (1975). The effects of videotaped modeling and confrontation on the drinking behavior of alcoholics. *International Journal of the Addictions, 10,* 779–793.

Baldwin, S., Heather, N., Lawson, A., et al. (1991). Comparison of effectiveness: Behavioral and talk-based alcohol education courses for court-
referred young offenders. *Behavioural Psychotherapy, 19*, 157–172.

Ball, S. A., Todd, M., Tennen, H., et al. (2007). Brief motivational enhancement and coping skills interventions for heavy drinking. *Addictive Behaviors, 32*(6), 1105–1118.

Brown, R. A. (1980). Conventional education and controlled drinking education courses with convicted drunken drivers. *Behavior Therapy, 11*,
632–642.

Caddy, G. R., & Lovibond, S. H. (1976). Self-regulation and discriminated
aversive conditioning in the modification of alcoholics' drinking behavior. *Behavior Therapy, 7*, 223–230.

Carpenter, R. A., Lyons, C. A., & Miller, W. R. (1985). Peer-managed self-
control program for prevention of alcohol abuse in American Indian
high school students: A pilot evaluation study. *International Journal of the
Addictions, 20*, 299–310.

Coghlan, G. R. (1979). *The investigation of behavioral self-control theory and
techniques in a short-term treatment of male alcohol abusers.* (MI No.
7918818). Unpublished doctoral dissertation, State University of New
York at Albany.

Connors, G. J., Tarbox, A. R., & Faillace, L. A. (1992). Achieving and maintaining gains among problem drinkers: Process and outcome results.
Behavior Therapy, 23, 449–474.

Connors, G. J., & Walitzer, K. S. (2001). Reducing alcohol consumption
among heavily drinking women: Evaluating the contributions of life-
skills training and booster sessions. *Journal of Consulting and Clinical Psychology, 69*(3), 447–456.

Copeland, L. A., Blow, F. C., & Barry, K. L. (2003). Health care utilization
by older alcohol-using veterans: Effects of a brief intervention to reduce
at-risk drinking. *Health Education and Behavior, 30*(3), 305–321.

Foy, D. W., Nunn, B. L., & Rychtarik, R. G. (1984). Broad-spectrum behavioral treatment for chronic alcoholics: Effects of training controlled
drinking skills. *Journal of Consulting and Clinical Psychology, 52*, 213–
230.

Graber, R. A., & Miller, W. R. (1988). Abstinence or controlled drinking
goals for problem drinkers: A randomized clinical trial. *Psychology of
Addictive Behaviors, 2*, 20–33.

Guydish, J. R. (1987). *Self-control bibliotherapy as a secondary prevention strategy with heavy-drinking college students.* Unpublished doctoral dissertation, Washington State University.

Harris, K. B., & Miller, W. R. (1990). Behavioral self-control training for problem drinkers: Components of efficacy. *Psychology of Addictive Behaviors,
4*, 82–90.

Heather, N., Brodie, J., Wale, S., et al. (2000). A randomized controlled trial of moderation-oriented cue exposure. *Journal of Studies on Alcohol and Drugs, 61*(4), 561–570.

Hester, R. K., & Delaney, H. D. (1997). Behavioral self-control program for Windows: Results of a controlled clinical trial. *Journal of Consulting and Clinical Psychology, 65*, 686–693.

Hester, R. K., Delaney, H. D., Campbell, W., et al. (2009). A web application for moderation training: Initial results of a randomized clinical trial. *Journal of Substance Abuse Treatment, 37*(3), 266–276.

Kennedy, P. J. (1989). *The effect of moderate drinking skill training on alcohol-related knowledge, attitude, and behavior.* Unpublished doctoral dissertation, University of Minnesota.

Kivlahan, D. R., Marlatt, G. A., Fromme, K., et al. (1990). Secondary prevention with college drinkers: Evaluation of an alcohol skills training program. *Journal of Consulting and Clinical Psychology, 58*, 805–810.

Koerkel, J. (2006). Behavioral self-management with problem drinkers: One-year follow-up of a controlled drinking group treatment approach. *Addiction Research and Theory, 14*(1), 35–49.

Lovibond, S. H. (1975). Use of behavior modification in the reduction of alcohol-related road accidents. In K. G. Götestam, G. L. Melin, & W. S. Dockens (Eds.), *Applications of behavior modification* (pp. 399–406). New York: Academic Press.

Marques, A. C. P. R., & Formigoni, M. L. O. S. (2001). Comparison of individual and group cognitive-behavioral therapy for alcohol and/or drug-dependent patients. *Addiction, 96*(6), 835–846.

Miller, W. R. (1978). Behavioral treatment of problem drinkers: A comparative outcome study of three controlled drinking therapies. *Journal of Consulting and Clinical Psychology, 46*, 74–86.

Miller, W. R., & Baca, L. M. (1983). Two-year follow-up of bibliotherapy and therapist-directed controlled drinking training for problem drinkers. *Behavior Therapy, 14*, 441–448.

Miller, W. R., Gribskov, C. J., & Mortell, R. L. (1981). Effectiveness of a self-control manual for problem drinkers with and without therapist contact. *International Journal of the Addictions, 16*, 1247–1254.

Miller, W. R., Leckman, A. L., Delaney, H. D., et al. (1992). Long-term follow-up of behavioral self-control training. *Journal of Studies on Alcohol, 53*, 249–261.

Miller, W. R., & Taylor, C. A. (1980). Relative effectiveness of bibliotherapy, individual and group self-control training in the treatment of problem drinkers. *Addictive Behaviors, 5*, 13–24.

Miller, W. R., Taylor, C. A., & West, J. C. (1980). Focused versus broad-spectrum behavior therapy for problem drinkers. *Journal of Consulting and Clinical Psychology, 48*, 590–601.

Morgenstern, J., Irwin, T. W., Wainberg, M. L., et al. (2007). A randomized controlled trial of goal choice interventions for alcohol use disorders among men who have sex with men. *Journal of Consulting and Clinical Psychology, 75*(1), 72–84.

Pomerleau, O., Pertschuk, M., Adkins, D., et al. (1978). A comparison of behavioral and traditional treatment for middle-income problem drinkers. *Journal of Behavioral Medicine, 1,* 187–200.

Riper, H., Kramer, J., Smit, F., et al. (2008). Web-based self-help for problem drinkers: A pragmatic randomized trial. *Addiction, 103*(2), 218–227.

Robertson, I., Heather, N., Dzialdowski, A., et al. (1986). A comparison of minimal versus intensive controlled drinking treatment for problem drinkers. *British Journal of Clinical Psychology, 25,* 185–194.

Sanchez-Craig, M., Annis, H. M., Bornet, A. R., et al. (1984). Random assignment to abstinence and controlled drinking: Evaluation of a cognitive-behavioural program for problem drinkers. *Journal of Consulting and Clinical Psychology, 52,* 390–403.

Sanchez-Craig, M., Leigh, G., Spivak, K., et al. (1989). Superior outcome of females over males after brief treatment for the reduction of heavy drinking. *British Journal of Addiction, 84,* 395–404.

Sanchez-Craig, M., Spivak, K., & Davila, R. (1991). Superior outcome of females over males after brief treatment for the reduction of heavy drinking: Replication and report of therapist effects. *British Journal of Addiction, 86,* 867–876.

Sandahl, C., & Ronnberg, S. (1990). Brief group psychotherapy relapse prevention for alcohol dependent patients. *International Journal of Group Psychotherapy, 40,* 453–476.

Skutle, A., & Berg, G. (1987). Training in controlled drinking for early-stage problem drinkers. *British Journal of Addiction, 82,* 493–501.

Sobell, M. B., & Sobell, L. C. (1973). Individualized behavior therapy for alcoholics. *Behavior Therapy, 4,* 49–72.

Spivak, K., Sanchez-Craig, M., & Davila, R. (1994). Assisting problem drinkers to change on their own: Effect of specific and non-specific advice. *Addiction, 89,* 1135–1142.

Vogler, R. E., Weissbach, T. A., Compton, J. V., et al. (1977). Integrated behavior change techniques for problem drinkers in the community. *Journal of Consulting and Clinical Psychology, 45*(2), 267–279.

Walitzer, K. S., & Connors, G. J. (2007). Thirty-month follow-up of drinking moderation training for women: A randomized clinical trial. *Journal of Consulting and Clinical Psychology, 75*(3), 501–507.

Other Self-Help Resources Based on a Moderation Goal

Although the program in this book was the first one published on behavioral self-control for moderation (*How to Control Your Drinking*, Miller & Muñoz,

1976), we wish to acknowledge that many other self-help guides for drinkers have been published over the decades. Here are some of them. Of these, only the books by Nick Heather and by Martha Sanchez-Craig have been tested for their effectiveness as self-help resources.

Amit, Z., Sutherland, E. A., & Weiner, A. (1977). *Guide to intelligent drinking.* New York: Walker & Company.

Dimeff, L. A., Baer, J. S., Kivlahan, D. R., et al. (1999). *Brief Alcohol Screening and Intervention for College Students (BASICS): A harm reduction approach.* New York: Guilford Press.

Heather, N., Richmond, R., Webster, I., et al. (1989). *A guide to healthier drinking: A self-help manual.* Sydney, Australia: Clarendon.

Miller, P. M. (1978). *Personal habit control.* New York: Simon & Schuster.

Robertson, I., & Heather, N. (1999). *So you want to cut down on your drinking?* Edinburgh: Health Education Board for Scotland.

Rotgers, F., et al. (2002). *Responsible drinking: A moderation management approach for problem drinkers.* Oakland, CA: New Harbinger.

Sanchez-Craig, M. (1993). *DrinkWise: How to quit drinking or cut down.* Toronto: Addiction Research Foundation.

Vogler, R. E., & Bartz, W. R. (1982). *The better way to drink.* New York: Simon & Schuster.

Williams, R. L., & Long, J. D. (1979). All things in moderation: Controlled drinking. In *Toward a self-managed life style* (2nd ed.). Boston: Houghton Mifflin.

Scholarly Reviews and Critiques of Self-Control and Moderation

There is a large and complex scientific literature on self-regulation and addictive behaviors. Beyond reading the original studies, there are summaries and commentaries on research in this area. These offer the advantage of drawing together a large body of research in a more understandable format.

Baumeister, R. F., Heatherton, T. F., & Tice, D. M. (1994). *Losing control: How and why people fail at self-regulation.* San Diego: Academic Press.

Fingarette, H. (1988). *Heavy drinking: The myth of alcoholism as a disease.* Berkeley and Los Angeles: University of California Press.

Heather, N., & Robertson, I. (1981). *Controlled drinking.* New York: Methuen.

Hester, R. K. (2003). Behavioral self-control training. In R. K. Hester & W. R. Miller (Eds.), *Handbook of alcoholism treatment approaches: Effective alternatives* (3rd ed., pp. 152–164). Boston: Allyn & Bacon.

Logue, A. W. (1995). *Self-control.* Englewood Cliffs, NJ: Prentice Hall.

Marlatt, G. A., & Witkiewitz, K. (2002). Harm reduction approaches to alcohol use: Health promotion, prevention, and treatment. *Addictive Behaviors, 27*(6), 867–886.

Miller, W. R. (1983). Controlled drinking: A history and critical review. *Journal of Studies on Alcohol, 44,* 68–83.

Peele, S. (1985). *The meaning of addiction: Compulsive experience and its interpretation.* Lexington, MA: Lexington Books.

Saladin, M. E., & Santa Ana, E. J. (2004). Controlled drinking: More than just a controversy. *Current Opinion in Psychiatry, 17*(3), 175–187.

Sobell, M. B., & Sobell, L. C. (1993). *Problem drinkers: Guided self-change treatment.* New York: Guilford Press.

Vaillant, G. E. (1995). *The natural history of alcoholism revisited.* Cambridge, MA: Harvard University Press.

Walters, G. D. (2000). Behavioral self-control training for problem drinkers: A meta-analysis of randomized control studies. *Behavior Therapy, 31*(1), 135–149.

Witkiewitz, K., & Marlatt, G. A. (2006). Overview of harm reduction treatments for alcohol problems. *International Journal of Drug Policy, 17*(4), 285–294.

Zinberg, N. E. (1984). *Drug, set, and setting: The basis for controlled intoxicant use.* New Haven, CT: Yale University Press.

Index

Abstinence. *See also* Quitting drinking
determining if its warranted, 9–10,
21–22
health problems associated with heavy
drinking and, 243–246
moderation attempts and, 16
overview, 231–233
pros and cons to, 11–15
Abstinence syndrome, 33
Acceptance, mindfulness and, 187–188
Acceptance and commitment therapy
(ACT), 199
Activities linked to drinking, 123–124,
149–154. *See also* Triggers
Addiction
dependent drinking and, 8
overview, 33
taking a vacation from alcohol and, 32
Aggression, 204–208
Aging, 244–245
Alcohol abuse. *See* Harmful drinking
Alcohol availability. *See* Availability of
money or alcohol
Alcohol Dependence Scale (ADS), 24–29
"Alcoholic" label, 4, 8–9, 225–226
Alcoholics Anonymous (AA), 234–235,
273–274
Alcohol-related problems, 249–250. *See
also* Effects of drinking
Amounts when drinking, 3, 9. *See
also* Dependent drinking; Dumb
drinking; Harmful drinking;
Overdrinking
Anger, 117–118, 203–204
Anxiety. *See also* Feelings; Stress
acceptance and commitment therapy
(ACT) and, 199
coping desensitization and, 197–198
dealing with unpleasant memories,
200–202

desensitization techniques, 195–199
exposure and response prevention
therapy and, 198–199
live desensitization and, 198
overview, 115–117, 193–195, 247
relaxation and, 135–136
systematic desensitization and, 195–
197
Assertiveness, 203–208. *See also*
Communication
Availability of money or alcohol, 102, 113,
114. *See also* Triggers
Awareness, 186–187

B

Bars. *See* Places that trigger more alcohol
consumption
Behavior
abstinence and, 22
acting "as if," 218–222
assertiveness and, 204–208
personal reality and, 132–134
pleasant activities without alcohol,
150–154
social skills and, 213
Beliefs, 133
Blood alcohol concentration (BAC)
estimating your BAC level, 44–47,
251–267
knowing from bodily sensations, 47
limit setting with drinking and, 49–54
overview, 40–47
slowing down alcohol consumption
and, 76
sobering up and, 47–49
tables for estimating, 251–267
types of drinks, 71–72
Body scan, 189–190
Boredom, 122–123
Brain functioning, 244–245

Breath exercises. *See also* Relaxation
    mindfulness meditation, 189
    overview, 138–139
    SOBER breathing space, 190

C

Cardiovascular system, 245–246
Center for Epidemiological Studies—
    Depression Scale (CES-D), 158,
    160–161
Central nervous system, 244–245
Change, 67–69
Choice, pros and cons to drinking and,
    230–231
Cigarette smoking, 97, 122
Cognitive-behavioral therapy (CBT), 236
Communication. *See also* Relationships
    assertiveness and, 203–208
    conflict and, 214–217
    overview, 209
    self-talk and, 146–147
    social skills and, 212–214
Community reinforcement approach
    (CRA), 235–236
Conflict, 118–119, 214–217
Control
    abstinence and, 22
    pros and cons to drinking and, 230–231
Coping desensitization, 197–198. *See also*
    Desensitization
Coping skills, 236
Counseling. *See* Professional help
Cutting back on drinking, 11–15. *See also*
    Moderation

D

Daily limits, recommended, 36–37. *See also*
    Limit setting with drinking
Daily Record Cards. *See also* Self-
    monitoring
    how long to use, 96
    situations in which you drink and,
        102–103, 126–127
Date rape, 7
Days of week for drinking, 101, 112–114.
    See also Situations in which you
    drink; Triggers
Dependency, 33. *See also* Addiction
Dependent drinking. *See also* Dumb
    drinking; Harmful drinking;
    Overdrinking
    overview, 3–4, 8
    self-evaluations regarding, 22–28, 29
    withdrawal symptoms and, 129–130
Depression. *See also* Feelings
    connection between drinking, mood,
        and, 161–163
    managing your mood, 163–166

overview, 118, 155–156, 165–166
    pleasant activities and, 150
    screening and, 156–161
    suicidal ideas and, 166–167
Desensitization
    coping desensitization, 197–198
    exposure and response prevention
        therapy, 198–199
    live desensitization, 198
    systematic desensitization, 195–197
    tips for, 199
Detoxification programs, 241. *See also*
    Professional help
Diagnosis, 22, 156, 159
Disappointment, 118
Disease. *See* Health problems
Drinks. *See also* Limit setting with
    drinking
    defining what constitutes a "drink,"
        35–36
    making drinks last longer, 72–74
    national average, 37–39
    self-monitoring and, 57–59
    spacing, 74–78
    types of, 71–72
Driving
    abstinence and, 22
    dumb drinking and, 6–7
Dumb drinking, 3–4, 6–7, 22–28, 29. *See
    also* Dependent drinking; Harmful
    drinking; Overdrinking

E

Eating, 49, 191–192
Effects of drinking. *See also* Health
    problems; Impairment; Intoxicating
    effects of alcohol
    blood alcohol concentration (BAC)
        and, 40–47
    dealing with unpleasant memories and,
        200
    fear and anxiety and, 194
    feelings and, 116–117
    health problems associated with heavy
        drinking, 243–246
    list of alcohol-related problems, 249–250
    mental health, 247
    overview, 19, 129–130
    personal abilities, 130–132
    personal reality and, 132–134
    relaxation, 135–136
    sleep and, 178–179
    sobering up and, 47–49
    social functioning, 247
    spirituality, 246–247
Emotions. *See* Feelings
Encouragement, 83–85, 143–148
Endocrine systems, 246

Equanimity, 187–188. *See also* Mindfulness
Expectations
     forming friendships and, 211
     personal reality and, 133
Expectations regarding this program,
     16–18
Exposure techniques, 198–199

F
Fear. *See also* Anxiety; Feelings
     acceptance and commitment therapy
          (ACT) and, 199
     coping desensitization and, 197–198
     dealing with unpleasant memories,
          200–202
     desensitization techniques, 195–199
     exposure and response prevention
          therapy and, 198–199
     live desensitization and, 198
     overview, 193–195
     systematic desensitization and, 195–197
Feedback regarding your drinking, 55. *See
     also* Self-monitoring
Feelings. *See also* Anxiety; Depression;
          Fear; Mood effects; Triggers
     anxiety and stress, 115–117
     assertiveness and, 206–207
     conflict, 118–119
     connection between drinking, mood,
          and depression, 161–163
     depression and disappointment, 118
     frustration and anger, 117–118
     managing your mood, 163–166
     overview, 102, 115, 119
     personal reality and, 132–134
     pleasant activities without alcohol,
          150–154
     screening and, 156–161
     self-concept and, 168–169
     self-talk and, 143–148
Friends. *See also* People who trigger more
          alcohol consumption; Relationships
     conflict and, 118–119, 214–217
     forming friendships, 210–212
     pros and cons to drinking and, 228–230
     refusing drinks and, 79–82
     support from, 91–94
Frustration, 117–118, 203–204
Fun, 218–222. *See also* Activities linked to
     drinking; Pleasant activities without
     alcohol

G
Gastrointestinal system, 245
Goals
     blood alcohol concentration (BAC)
          and, 40–47
     examples of, 50–54

limit setting with drinking, 35–40,
     49–54
overview, 9–10
personal reality and, 133–134
reasons to continue or cut back on/quit
     drinking, 11–15
rewarding and encouraging yourself
     and, 83–94
self-concept and, 173–176
Gradual approach, 195–197

H
Habits, 67–69, 233
Harmful drinking. *See also* Dependent
          drinking; Dumb drinking;
          Overdrinking
     health problems associated with, 243–246
     overview, 3–4, 7–8
     recommended daily limits to avoid,
          36–37
     self-evaluations regarding, 22–28, 29,
          249–250
Health problems. *See also* Effects of
          drinking
     abstinence and, 22
     associated with heavy drinking,
          243–246
     pros and cons to drinking and, 226–227
     risks of involved with overdrinking, 5
Healthy management of reality, 132–134,
     221
Heart functioning, 245–246
Help, professional. *See* Professional help
Holiday heart syndrome, 246
Hormonal functioning, 246
Hunger, 102, 121–122. *See also* Triggers

I
Illness. *See* Health problems
Immune system, 245
Impairment. *See also* Effects of drinking;
          Intoxicating effects of alcohol
     blood alcohol concentration (BAC)
          and, 40–47
     dumb drinking and, 6–7
     sobering up and, 47–49
Inactivity, 122–123
Inpatient treatment programs, 241. *See also*
     Professional help
Insomnia. *See* Sleeping well
Intelligence, 244–245
Intensive outpatient treatment programs,
     241. *See also* Professional help
Intoxicating effects of alcohol. *See also*
          Effects of drinking; Impairment
     blood alcohol concentration (BAC)
          and, 40–47
     sobering up and, 47–49

J

Judgment impairment, 41–43. *See also* Effects of drinking; Impairment

L

Labels, 4, 8–9, 225–226
Leisure activities. *See* Activities linked to drinking; Pleasant activities without alcohol
Limit setting with drinking. *See also* Moderation; Triggers
    blood alcohol concentration (BAC) and, 40–47
    days and times you drink and, 112–114
    defining what constitutes a "drink," 35–36
    estimating your BAC level, 45–46
    examples of, 50–54
    national average, 37–39
    overview, 35–40, 49–54
    recommended daily limits, 36–37
    refusing drinks, 79–82
    rewarding and encouraging yourself and, 83–94
    situations in which you drink and, 127–128
    slowing down alcohol consumption, 70–78
    sobering up and, 47–49
    support from others and, 91–94
Live desensitization, 198. *See also* Desensitization
Liver, 245

M

Medical conditions. *See* Health problems
Medication use
    abstinence and, 22
    to help you quit drinking, 237–238
    increasing as you decrease alcohol use, 97
Meditation. *See* Mindfulness
Memories, 200–202
Mental abilities, 244–245
Mental health, 247, 270–272
Methods, 18–19, 67–69. *See also individual methods*
Michigan Alcoholism Screening Test (MAST), 22–24, 27–28, 29
Mindfulness. *See also* Relaxation
    benefits of, 185–188
    examples of, 184–185
    mindfulness meditation, 187, 188–192
Mindfulness-based cognitive therapy (MBCT), 185–186
Mindfulness-based relapse prevention (MBRP), 185–186

Mindfulness-based stress reduction (MBSR), 185–186
Moderation. *See also* Cutting back on drinking; Limit setting with drinking
    Alcoholics Anonymous (AA) and, 273–274
    blood alcohol concentration (BAC) and, 40–47
    choosing abstinence and, 231–233
    determining if it's warranted, 10
    limit setting with drinking, 35–40
    overview, 225–226
    people who trigger, 110–111
    places that trigger, 106–107
    pros and cons to, 11–15, 226–231
    research on, 20–22
    self-evaluations regarding, 22–28, 29
    self-management toolbox and, 18–19
    situations in which you drink and, 127–128
    sobering up and, 49
    spacing drinks and, 75
    support from others and, 91–94
    transitioning to, 32
    working through this program and, 15–18
Money availability. *See* Availability of money or alcohol
Mood disorders, 247. *See also* Anxiety; Depression
Mood effects. *See also* Depression; Effects of drinking; Feelings
    blood alcohol concentration (BAC) and, 40–47
    connection between drinking, mood, and depression, 161–163
    managing your mood, 163–166
    pleasant activities without alcohol, 150–154
    screening and, 156–161
Mood Screener
    complete, 157
    diagnosis and, 156
    overview, 159–160
Motivational interviewing (MI), 236–237
Muscle relaxation, 137–138. *See also* Relaxation

N

Negative feelings, 206–207. *See also* Feelings
Negative moods. *See* Depression; Feelings; Mood effects
Negative thoughts, 172–173. *See also* Self-talk; Thoughts
Negotiations, 215–217

O

Outpatient treatment programs, 241. *See also* Professional help
Overdrinking. *See also* Dependent drinking; Dumb drinking; Harmful drinking
as a habit, 32
health problems associated with, 243–246
overview, 3–6
people who trigger, 109–110
places that trigger, 105–106
self-evaluations regarding, 22–28, 29
situations in which you drink and, 105–106, 109–110, 131–132
slowing down alcohol consumption and, 76
Over-the-counter medicines. *See* Medication use

P

Pain, 117
Partners. *See* Support from others
Passive behavior, 204–208
Payday, 113, 114
People who trigger more alcohol consumption, 101, 108–111. *See also* Friends; Situations in which you drink; Triggers
Perfectionism
self-concept and, 175–176
working through this program and, 17–18
Personal Goals Card, 49–50
Personal reality, 132–134
Physical dependence, 130. *See also* Dependent drinking
Physical health. *See* Health problems
Places that trigger more alcohol consumption, 101, 104–107. *See also* Situations in which you drink; Triggers
Planning ahead
pleasant activities without alcohol, 154
self-talk and, 145–146
sleep and, 179–180
Pleasant activities without alcohol, 149
Positive effects of drinking. *See* Effects of drinking
Positive feelings, 206–207. *See also* Feelings
Positive thoughts, 169–173. *See also* Self-talk; Thoughts
Pregnancy, 21–22, 247
Problem drinking. *See* Harmful drinking
Professional help
choosing abstinence and, 232
community reinforcement approach (CRA), 235–236
coping skills, 236
fear and anxiety and, 198–199
medications, 237–238
mindfulness-based approaches, 185–186
motivational interviewing (MI), 236–237
overview, 234, 238–241, 241–242
sleep and, 183
social anxiety and, 209
suicidal ideas and, 166–167
treatment settings, 241
12-step programs, 234–235
Progress summary, 64–66, 83–94
Progressive deep muscle relaxation, 136, 137–138, 190. *See also* Relaxation
Pros and cons to drinking
choosing abstinence and, 231–233
overview, 11–15, 226–231
Psychological dependence, 130. *See also* Dependent drinking

Q

Quitting drinking, 11–15, 231–233. *See also* Abstinence

R

Rate of drinking
changing, 19
places and, 104
rapid-paced drinking, 7
Reality, personal. *See* Personal reality
Reducing drinking. *See* Cutting back on drinking
Refusing drinks
assertiveness and, 204–205
overview, 79–82
people who trigger overdrinking and, 109–110
Relapse prevention, 236
Relationships. *See also* Communication; Friends; Support from others
assertiveness and, 203–208
conflict and, 118–119, 214–217
forming, 210–212
overview, 209
pros and cons to drinking and, 228–230
self-talk and, 146–147
social skills and, 212–214
Relaxation. *See also* Mindfulness
breath exercises, 138–139
as a goal of drinking, 115–117
overview, 135–136
progressive deep muscle relaxation, 137–138
sleep and, 179, 182
systematic desensitization and, 195–197

Relaxation (*cont.*)
    techniques for and their applications,
        137–142
    visual images for relaxing, 139–140
Religious beliefs, 235, 246–247
Resisting drinks offered, 79–82
Resources, 269–272
Response prevention therapy, 198–199
Restaurants. *See* Places that trigger more
        alcohol consumption
Rewarding yourself
    "congratulations" agreement, 89–90
    examples of, 89–90
    ideas for rewards, 86–89
    overview, 83–85
    resistance to the idea of, 85
    support from others and, 91–94
Risk taking. *See also* Effects of drinking;
        Impairment
    blood alcohol concentration (BAC)
        and, 43
    dumb drinking and, 7

S

Safety, 6–7
Scheduling. *See* Planning ahead
Screening
    Center for Epidemiological Studies—
        Depression Scale (CES-D), 158,
        160–161
    depression and negative moods, 156–161
    list of alcohol-related problems, 249–250
    Mood Screener, 157, 159–160
    overview, 22
Sedatives. *See* Medication use
Self-concept
    overview, 168–169
    self-thoughts and, 169–173
    setting standards for yourself and,
        173–176
Self-control approach
    examples of, 50–54
    overview, 95–98
    self-evaluations regarding, 22–28
    situations in which you drink and,
        127–128
    taking a vacation from alcohol and, 32
Self-esteem, 168, 169
Self-evaluations, 22–28, 29, 223–224,
        225–233. *See also* Mood Screener;
        Center for Epidemiological Studies—
        Depression Scale (CES-D)
Self-management toolbox, 18–19, 67–69.
        See also individual methods
Self-monitoring
    connection between drinking, mood,
        and depression, 161–163
    examples of, 62–64, 65–66

explaining to others when asked, 60–64
    overview, 55–57
    rewarding and encouraging yourself
        and, 89
    self-monitoring cards, 57–60
    steps for, 62
    summary of progress, 64–66
Self-talk
    managing your mood, 164–165
    overview, 143–148
    self-concept and, 169–173
Sex differences
    estimating your BAC level, 44, 45–46
    limit setting with drinking and, 37
    national average, 37–39
    slowing down alcohol consumption
        and, 76
Sexual experiences, 120
Sickness. *See* Health problems
Sipping, 72–74
Situations in which you drink. *See
        also* Days of week for drinking;
        People who trigger more alcohol
        consumption; Places that trigger
        more alcohol consumption; Time of
        day for drinking; Triggers
    effects of drinking and, 131–132
    overview, 19, 101–103, 126–128
    self-talk and, 145
Sleeping pills. *See* Medication use
Sleeping well
    effects of drinking and, 178–179
    nightmares, 183
    overview, 177–178
    sleep and, 179–181
    waking up at night, 181–183
Slowing down alcohol consumption
    making drinks last longer, 72–74
    overview, 70
    refusing drinks and, 79–82
    spacing drinks, 74–78
    types of drinks, 71–72
Slowing down your drinking. *See* Rate of
        drinking
Smoking, 97, 122
SOBER breathing space, 190. *See also*
        Breath exercises
Sobering up, 47–49
Social functioning, 247
Social skills, 212–214, 228–230. *See also*
        Communication
Socializing. *See also* Communication;
        Relationships
    forming friendships, 210–212
    overview, 209
    pros and cons to drinking and, 228–
        230
Spirituality, 235, 246–247

Spouses, 91–94
Standard drink. *See* Drinks
Standards for yourself, 173–176
Stress, 115–117, 135–142, 193–195. *See also* Anxiety
Substance use (other than alcohol). *See* Medication use; Tobacco use
Suicidal ideas, 166–167, 247
Summary of Progress form, 64–66, 83
Support from others. *See also* Friends; Relationships
  examples of, 93–94
  people who trigger overdrinking and, 110
  rewarding and encouraging yourself and, 91–94
Symptoms of withdrawal. *See* Withdrawal symptoms
Systematic desensitization, 195–197. *See also* Desensitization

T

Tension, 135–136, 193–194. *See also* Anxiety; Stress
Therapy. *See* Professional help
Thirst, 102, 121. *See also* Triggers
Thought stopping method, 172–173
Thoughts. *See also* Feelings
  acting "as if," 219–220
  connection between drinking, mood, and depression, 161–163
  dealing with unpleasant memories, 200–202
  managing your mood, 163–166
  personal reality and, 132–134
  self-concept and, 168–173
  self-talk and, 143–148
Time of day for drinking, 101, 112–114. *See also* Situations in which you drink; Triggers
Tobacco use, 97, 122

Tolerance
  estimating your BAC level, 47, 48
  slowing down alcohol consumption and, 70
Tracking your drinking. *See* Self-monitoring
Tranquilizers. *See* Medication use
Treatment. *See* Professional help
Triggers. *See also* Situations in which you drink
  days and times, 112–114
  effects of drinking and, 131
  feelings, 115–119
  hunger, 121–122
  identifying, 101–103
  inactivity, 122–123
  overview, 19, 99, 120, 126–128
  particular activities, 123–124
  people, 108–111
  places, 104–107
  smoking, 122
  thirst, 121
  tips for dealing with, 124–125
Turning down drinks
  assertiveness and, 204–205
  overview, 79–82
  people who trigger overdrinking and, 109–110
12-step programs, 234–235, 273–274

U

Urge surfing, 191

V

Vacation from alcohol, 32
Violence, 7, 22
Visualization exercises, 139–140, 191. *See also* Relaxation

W

Withdrawal symptoms, 8, 33, 129–130

About the Authors

William R. Miller, PhD, is Emeritus Distinguished Professor of Psychology and Psychiatry at the University of New Mexico. He has published over 400 scientific articles and chapters and more than 40 books, including the groundbreaking work for professionals *Motivational Interviewing.* Fundamentally interested in the psychology of change, Dr. Miller has focused particularly on developing and testing more effective treatments for people with alcohol and drug problems. The Institute for Scientific Information lists him as one of the world's most cited scientists.

Ricardo F. Muñoz, PhD, is Distinguished Professor of Clinical Psychology at Palo Alto University and Emeritus Professor of Psychology at the University of California, San Francisco. His major areas of expertise include addictive behavior, the prevention and treatment of depression, and how depression affects substance use. He has published over 100 scientific articles and chapters and several books, including *Control Your Depression* and *The Prevention of Depression.*